Questions and Answers

2nd Edition

Volume 2

By Stu Silverstein, M.D., FAAP

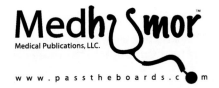

www.passtheboards.com

MedHumor Medical Publications, Stamford, Connecticut

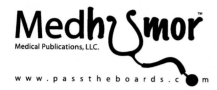

www.passtheboards.com

Published by:
    Medhumor Medical Publications, LLC
    1127 High Ridge Road, Suite 332
    Stamford, CT 06905 U.S.A.

Copyright © 2002, 2008 Medhumor Medical Publications, LLC

ISBN: **0-9771374-9-X**

First Edition Copyright © 2002 Medhumor Medical Publications, LLC
Second Edition Copyright © 2008 Medhumor Medical Publications, LLC

Printed in the United States of America .

This book is designed to provide information and guidance in regard to the subject matter covered. It is to be used as a study guide for physicians preparing for the General Pediatric Certifying Exam administered by the American Board of Pediatrics. It is not meant to be a clinical manual. The reader is advised to consult textbooks and other reference manuals in making clinical decisions. It is not the purpose of this book to reprint all the information that is otherwise available, but rather to assist the Board Candidate in organizing the material to facilitate study and recall on the exam. The reader is encouraged to read other sources of material, in particular picture atlases that are available.

Although every precaution has been taken in the preparation of this book, the publisher, author, and members of the editorial board assume no responsibility for errors, omissions or typographical mistakes. Neither is any liability assumed for damages resulting from the direct and indirect use of the information contained herein. The book contains information that is up-to-date only up to the printing date. Due to the very nature of the medical profession, there will be points out-of-date as soon as the book rolls off the press. The purpose of this book is to educate and entertain.

**If you do not wish to be bound by the above,
you may return this book to the publisher for a full refund.**

Publisher:	MedHumor Medical Publications, LLC Stamford, CT
VP/Content Development :	Stuart Silverstein, MD, FAAP Clinical Director Firefly After Hours Pediatrics, LLC Stamford, CT Assistant Clinical Professor Emergency Medicine New York Medical College
Senior Editor:	Jon Durica, MD Stamford, CT
General Manager/ Operations:	Todd Van Allen
Design / Copy Editor:	Antoinette D'Amore, A.D. Design www.addesign-graphics.com
Cover Designer:	Rachel Mindrup www.rmindrup.com

About the Author

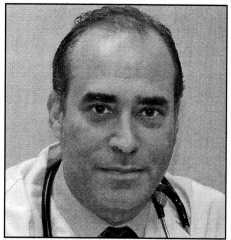

Dr. Stu Silverstein is the founder and CEO of Medhumor Medical Publications, LLC which began with the publication of the critically acclaimed "Laughing your way to Passing the Pediatric Boards"™ back in the spring of 2000. Word spread quickly that finally there was a book out there that turned a traditionally daunting process into one that was actually fun and enjoyable. This groundbreaking study guide truly "Took the Boredom out of Board review"® with reports from our readers that they were able to reduce their study and review time in half. Those who were taking the exam for the 2nd time not only passed but increased their scores dramatically.

Their supplementary pediatric titles have also been crtically acclaimed. Medhumor Publications LLC, has since expanded their catalogue to include a title for the USMLE Step 3 and the Neurolgy Board exams.

The concept of the "Laughing your way to Passing the Boards"™ and Medhumor Medical Publications, LLC were conceived by Dr. Silverstein. He brought his years of experience in the field of Standup Comedy and Comedy writing after he realized the critical need for a study guide that spoke the language of colleagues rather than the language of dusty textbooks. His work as a Standup Comedian and Medical Humorist has frequently been featured in several newspapers, radio programs and TV shows, including the New York Times, WCBS newsradio in NY City, as well as World News Tonight with Peter Jennings.

Dr. Silverstein has also served as a contributing editor for the <u>Resident and Staff Physician</u> annual board review issue and has authored numerous articles on medical humor. He has served on the faculty of the Osler Institute Board Review course, UCLA Pediatric Board Review course and several local board review courses. He is the co-author of "What about Me? Growing up with a Developmentally Disabled Sibling" written with Dr. Bryna Siegel, professor of Child Psychiatry , the University of California San Francisco. Dr. Silverstein is in demand as a lecturer for residency programs on successful preparation for the pediatric board exam.

In addition to writing, lecturing, and expanding the scope of Medhumor Medical Publications, LLC., Dr. Silverstein is the Clinical Director for Firefly After Hours Pediatrics, a subacute emergency practice. Dr. Silverstein is an Assistant Clinical Professor of Emergency Medicine at the New York Medical College in Valhalla, New York.

Questions and Answers Volume 2 (2nd Edition)

In putting together the 2nd edition of our *Question and Answer* series we did our utmost to incorporate the suggestions of our readers who successfully passed the General Pediatric Board Exam as well as the Recertification Exam.

Each book now contains 400 questions each broken down by subspecialty. This allows the reader to focus on areas that need improvement. Matching and questions based on clinical vignettes now count as one question. Therefore the 2nd edition contains significantly more questions than the 1st editions.

All questions have been reviewed and revised based on the content specifications published by the American Academy of Pediatrics. The infectious disease and preventive medicine questions were updated based on the most up to date information published in the online edition of the AAP "Red Book".

We hope that these updated *Question and Answer* books will continue to serve those for whom passing the pediatric certification and recertification exams is the next ticket to be punched.

—Stuart Silverstein, MD, FAAP
Stamford, CT

Table of Contents

Questions 1

Adolescent 3

Allergy & Immunology 6

Cardiology 9

Cognition, Language & Learning 18

Critical Care 20

Dermatology 22

Endocrinology 25

ENT 33

ER 39

Fluids & Lytes 47

Genetics 52

GI 57

GU 62

Heme Onc 64

ID 73

Metabolic 86

Musculoskeletal 89

Neonatology 94

Neurology 102

Nutrition 108

Pharmacology 112

Preventive 114

Psychosocial 118

Pulmonary 125

Renal 131

Rheumatology 136

Substance Abuse 139

Answers **141**

Adolescent 143

Allergy & Immunology 145

Cardiology 148

Cognition, Language & Learning 153

Critical Care 154

Dermatology 157

Endocrinology 159

ENT 165

ER 168

Fluids & Lytes 175

Genetics 178

GI 182

GU 186

Heme Onc 188

ID 195

Metabolic 204

Musculoskeletal 207

Neonatology 210

Neurology 217

Nutrition 222

Pharmacology 226

Preventive 227

Psychosocial 230

Pulmonary 236

Renal 240

Rheumatology 244

Substance Abuse 247

Icon Signposts

The question and answer sections contain an icon signpost indicating the significance of the highlighted material as follows:

PERIL ⚠ WARNING	*Perils*	This alerts you to possible big mistakes and traps that are typically laid down for you on the exam.

Questions

Adolescent

1) You are asked to medically clear a teenage female who is being admitted for anorexia nervosa who is currently 35% below ideal body weight. With regard to rapid refeeding which of the following should you be MOST concerned about? :

A) Hypokalemia
B) Hyperkalemia
C) Hyperphosphatemia
D) Hypophosphatemia
E) Hyponatremia

2) Which of one the following factors is MOST associated with early initiation of sexual activity in teenagers?

A) Higher socioeconomic status
B) Access to condoms in school based clinic
C) Sexual abuse
D) Late onset of puberty
E) Firm parental discipline at home

3) Which of the following is true regarding morbidity and mortality of teens?

A) Motor vehicle accidents are a leading cause of mortality but not morbidity in adolescents aged 16-20
B) For every adolescent killed in a motor vehicle accident 100 non fatal injuries occur
C) A 16 year old is twice as likely to have a crash while driving than the general population
D) The low morbidity of teens involved in motor vehicle accidents is due to their high rate of seat belt usage
E) Adolescents are immortal

4) **Which of the following should be kept in mind when counseling teenagers to not engage in high risk behavior?**

A) Adolescents have a high capacity for abstract thinking.
B) Long term impact of poor health habits are a strong deterrent
C) Linking cause and effect regarding health habits over several visits will gradually impact behavior
D) Reinforcing the impact the behavior will have on their appearance and physical performance compared with their peers should be emphasized
E) Have them sign a contract with their parents that they will refrain from high risk behavior

5) **Which of the following is true regarding sexual orientation in teenagers?**

A) Transient homosexual experimentation is uncommon
B) Adolescents who are emotionally attracted to members of the same gender usually engage in sexual activity
C) Adolescents struggling with issues of sexual preference should be discouraged from doing so
D) Approximately 30% of gay youths have attempted suicide at least once
E) Depression and suicide ideation are rare among homosexual teenagers

6) **Which of the following is true regarding scoliosis in teenagers?**

A) Scoliosis is by definition curvature of the spine greater than 15 degrees
B) Adolescent idiopathic scoliosis is defined as scoliosis whose onset is seen in children older than 15
C) Idiopathic scoliosis is more common in boys than girls
D) Mild – moderate pulmonary compromise can be seen in spine curvature greater than 60 degrees
E) Adolescent scoliosis is mostly associated with X-linked disorders

7) **Each of the following is a true statement regarding sexually transmitted diseases EXCEPT:**

A) Chlamydia trachomatis and Neisseria gonorrhea are often asymptomatic in males.
B) Chlamydia trachomatis and Neisseria gonorrhea are often asymptomatic in females.
C) 50% of sexually active adolescents become infected with sexually transmitted diseases each year.
D) Chronic pelvic pain can be a manifestation of PID
E) It is now possible to diagnose Chlamydia trachomatis and Neisseria gonorrhea using urine-based diagnostic testing

8)   Which of the following is true regarding noninvasive urine-based diagnostic testing?

A)   Females should obtain a sample from the first part of the stream without cleaning the perineum
B)   One urine sample to rule out urinary tract infection and a sexually transmitted disease is all that is necessary
C)   Urine amplification tests are acceptable evidence in abuse and assault cases
D)   Urine sampling is more sensitive but less specific than traditional culture-based testing
E)   Urine sampling is less sensitive but more specific

9)   Each of the following are significant considerations in the differential diagnosis of anovulatory uterine bleeding in an adolescent female, *except* :

A)   Hyperthyroidism
B)   Hypothyroidism
C)   Cystic fibrosis
D)   Hyperprolactinemia
E)   Ovarian failure

10) You are evaluating a 16 year old female who is new to your practice. She has been experiencing heavy, painless bleeding since the onset of menses. There is a significant family history for heavy menstrual bleeding in the family including the patient's mother. She is physically active, height and weight are both in the 60th percentile and her SMR is 5. The most likely explanation for the heavy menstrual bleeding would be:

A)   Factor VIII deficiency
B)   Factor IX deficiency
C)   Von Willebrand disease
D)   Polycystic ovary syndrome
E)   Crohn's disease

Allergy & Immunology

11) Match the immune response description on the left with the classified allergic reaction on the left.

1) Immune complex (Arthus reaction)
2) Delayed hypersensitivity
3) Anaphylactoid reaction
4) Antibody mediated

(A) Type 1 allergic reaction
(B) Type 2 allergic reaction
(C) Type 3 allergic reaction
(D) Type 4 allergic reaction

12) It's a Friday afternoon, the snow is blowing and the sun is setting, and you're thinking about the skiing trip you are headed for. "Doctor, we have a drop in 7 year old Sammy Snowster. He has fever and an earache." You glance at the problem list:

It's his ninth ear infection and each time he has had symptoms consistent with sinusitis.

In addition, he has had multiple episodes of bronchitis.

His immunizations are all up to date.

His physical exam is unremarkable except for the "I'm with Stupid" shirt he is wearing with the arrow pointed in your direction.

His CBC electrolytes and liver function tests have been consistently normal.

Your partner did check his hepatitis B titers, which were significantly low for someone who had completed his immunization set. You scratch your head, move out of the way so the arrow isn't pointed at you, and redeem yourself by making the following diagnosis:

A) Poor wardrobe. You replace his shirt with one that says "Don't Mess with Mr. Zero."
B) Just a poor response to the hepatitis B vaccine. After another full series, there should be no problem.
C) X-linked severe immunodeficiency.
D) Common variable immunodeficiency.
E) HIV. You start Bactrim prophylaxis and begin a full workup.

13) **Each of the following are associated with food allergy in children EXCEPT:**

A) High IgA in mother's colostrum
B) Early antigen exposure during the first few days of life
C) Positive family history of atopic disease
D) IgE mediated reactions
E) Food proteins found in breast milk that can serve as milk allergens

14) **A 6-month-old exclusively breast fed infant presents with a diffuse dry patchy, scaly erythematous skin rash worse on extensor surfaces. Itching is relieved partially with diphenhydramine. The MOST appropriate next step would be to:**

A) Switch to a soy based formula
B) Skin test the baby
C) Skin test the mother
D) Hydrocortisone 2% lotion
E) Order IgE levels on the baby

15) **The most frequent form of primary immunodeficiency is:**

A) Chronic granulomatous disease
B) AIDS
C) selective IgA deficiency
D) congenital X-linked agammaglobulinemia
E) hyperimmunoglobulin E syndrome

16) You are managing a patient in your practice who presents with failure to thrive, chronic diarrhea and candidal infections resistant to treatment. Lab results reveal hypocalcemia. Genetic studies reveal a hemizygous deletion of 22q11.2 You confirm that this child has DiGeorge Syndrome with significant T lymphocyte deficiency.

Which of the following options would be most appropriate in this patient?

A) Splenectomy
B) Bone marrow transplantation
C) Monthly T-lymphocyte replacement
D) Thymectomy
E) Thymic transplantation

17) Each of the following is true regarding X-linked hyper IgM syndrome *except* for:

A) Prophylaxis against P. jiroveci is indicated
B) Intravenous gammaglobulin treatment is indicated
C) IgG, IgA, IgE levels are low
D) IgM levels are elevated
E) IgG, IgA and IgE levels are elevated

18) Which of the following is true regarding IgA deficiency?

A) It is the least common primary immunodeficiency
B) Most patients with this defect have recurrent infections.
C) IgA deficiency is an indication for replacement immunoglobulin therapy
D) Circulating anti-IgA antibodies places patients at risk if transfused with immunoglobulin
E) Most asymptomatic cases have defects in one or more IgG subclasses

19) **Which of the following is true regarding the use of inhaled steroids in treating asthma?**

   A) They are risk-free
   B) On average adult height is 0.5 cm below expected
   C) Growth velocity is reduced during the first year of treatment
   D) Acne, mood swings and weight gain do not occur
   E) Oral candidiasis is the most rare complication

20) **Which of the following is the most appropriate treatment of chronic urticaria?**

   A) Topical diphenhydramine
   B) Topical hydrocortisone 2% lotion
   C) Hydroxyzine orally
   D) Diphenhydramine orally
   E) Fexofenadine orally

Cardiology

21) **All of the following are components of tetralogy of Fallot *EXCEPT* for:**

   A) Overriding aorta
   B) Pulmonary stenosis
   C) VSD
   D) Tricuspid atresia
   E) Right ventricular hypertrophy

22) Match each with the lettered choice that best corresponds to the EKG tracing.

(A)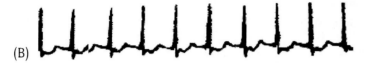

(B)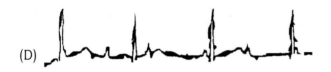

(C)

(D)

(E)

(F)

(G)

(H)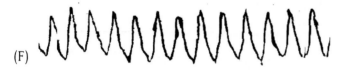

1) Ventricular Fibrillation (V-Fib)
2) Ventricular Tachycardia (V-Tach)
3) Wolf Parkinson White syndrome (WPW)
4) Sinus arrhythmia
5) 2nd degree AV block
6) 3rd degree AV block
7) Premature ventricular contraction (PVC)
8) Supraventricular tachycardia (SVT)

23) **Match the disease on the left with the murmur on the right.**

1) Aortic stenosis
2) Pulmonary stenosis
3) Coarctation of the aorta
4) ASD
5) VSD
6) PDA
7) Mitral insufficiency
8) Aortic insufficiency

(A) Abnormal fixed splitting of S2
(B) Diastolic decrescendo murmur
(C) Continuous murmur often heard best in the intraclavicular area
(D) Systolic ejection click that does not vary with respiration
(E) Presence of an ejection click that varies with respiration
(F) Holosystolic, or nearly so, and is heard best at the apex
(G) A continuous murmur over the back
(H) Diastolic rumble in mid-diastole, heard best along the lower left sternal border

24)   Each of the following is a cause of cyanotic heart disease in newborns EXCEPT:

A) d-Transposition of the great arteries
B) Truncus arteriosis
C) Aortic insufficiency
D) Tricuspid atresia
E) Anomalous (total) pulmonary venous return

25)   A 5-year-old child has a grade 2/6, mid-systolic, musical, medium-pitched cardiac murmur heard best along the left lower and midsternal border. Which of the following is the MOST likely diagnosis?

A) ASD
B) MVP
C) Innocent murmur
D) Pulmonary valve stenosis
E) VSD

26)   A left axis deviation is seen on EKG with all of the following EXCEPT:

A) Normal heart
B) AV canal defects
C) Tricuspid atresia
D) Double outlet right ventricle
E) Hypertrophic cardiomyopathy

27) An acyanotic 2-month-old boy is hospitalized because of irritability, poor feeding, and dyspnea of 7 days' duration. HR is 170/min, RR 60/min. Physical examination: harsh holosystolic murmur associated with a precordial systolic thrill at the lower left sternal border; there is a diastolic rumble at the apex.[1] Crackles are heard in both lung bases. The liver is palpable 3 cm below the right costal margin. Which of the following is the MOST likely diagnosis?

A) VSD
B) ASD
C) Complete transposition of the great arteries
D) Anomalous origin of the left coronary artery
E) TOF

28) During the transition from fetal circulation, the constriction of the patent ductus arteriosus and formation of the ligamentum arteriosum occur *primarily* because of:

A) Decreased PO2
B) Increased PO2
C) Decreased PCO2
D) Increased PCO2
E) None of the above

29) The gold standard for diagnosing *subacute bacterial endocarditis* would be:

A) Gold fillings during all dental procedures
B) A 24-hour EKG monitoring
C) Elevated white blood cell count with a left shift
D) A positive blood culture
E) Elevated erythrocyte sedimentation rate

---

[1] Are you ready to rumble?

30) The Cardiac cath oxygen saturation and pressure gradient demonstrated below is most consistent with:

A) Normal heart
B) Tetralogy of Fallot
C) Truncus arteriosis
D) Total anomalous venous return
E) Transposition of the great vessels

(SVC)	70%		98%		(PV)
(RA)	2 70%		5 98%		(LA)
(RV)	110/10 80%		110/10 80%		(LV)
Truncus	110/10 80%		110/10 80%		

31) **The Cardiac cath oxygen saturation and pressure gradient demonstrated below is most consistent with:**

A) Normal heart
B) Tetralogy of Fallot
C) Total anomalous venous return
D) Truncus arteriosis
E) Aortic stenosis

(SVC)	70%		95%	(PV)
(RA)	2		5	(LA)
	70%		95%	
(RV)	42/8		110/10	(LV)
	70%		75%	
PA	7		110/70	A
	70%		95%	

32) **The Cardiac cath oxygen saturation and pressure gradient demonstrated below is most consistent with:**

A) Normal heart
B) Tetralogy of Fallot
C) Total anomalous venous return
D) Pulmonary stenosis
E) Aortic stenosis

(SVC)	70%	95%	(PV)

(RA) 2 85%	(LA) 3 85%
(RV) 22/2 85%	(LV) 110/50 85%

PA	40/18 85%	110/50 85% A

33) **Which of the following is true regarding the management of cardiac complications of Kawasaki disease?**

A) High dose aspirin is given during the acute phase and then discontinued
B) Cardiac echo is done when Kawasaki is diagnosed to assess for coronary artery aneurysms
C) Cardiac complications include myocarditis and valvulitis
D) Low dose aspirin is given during the acute phase and then discontinued
E) Intravenous gamma globulin is given during the subacute phase

34) **You are evaluating a 16 year old varsity football player who is complaining of sharp left sided chest pain which increased with deep breaths. His grandfather died of a myocardial infarction at age 62 and his 57 year old father is being treated for hypertension. Physical examination is unremarkable**

The most appropriate next step in managing this patient is

A) Trial of antacids no restrictions on playing ball
B) Abdominal CT with IV contrast to assess for cholecystitis
C) Trial of ibuprofen and no restrictions
D) EKG if not ST changes clear for full activity
E) Cardiology referral and restriction of sports and other strenuous exercise

35) **Which of the following would be the most appropriate management of a child with a strong family history of familial hypercholesterolemia?**

A) Implement a low fat diet
B) Implement a low cholesterol diet
C) Measure serum triglycerides and cholesterol
D) Order a cardiac echo and stress test
E) Followup in 3 months after starting lipid lowering medications

Cognition, Language & Learning (Questions)

36) **With regards to learning disabilities in children, all of the following are true *EXCEPT* for which statement?**

   A) The most common learning disorders are developmental language disorders.
   B) Learning disabilities often coexist with other conditions such as anxiety and depression.
   C) Diagnosis is based on history and neuro-psychometric testing.
   D) A learning disability can coexist with an above average IQ.
   E) Most learning disabilities resolve by early adulthood.

37) **Each of the following represents a specific learning disability *EXCEPT* for:**

   A) Difficulties in reading
   B) Difficulties in writing
   C) Difficulties in math
   D) Difficulties in organizational skills
   E) Dyslexia

38) **During a routine physical you note that the child you are examining can walk upstairs with one hand held and turn the pages of your textbook 3 pages at a time. The parents tell you that he can speak 10 words and can identify 1 body part. The child's age is closest to:**

   A) 16 months
   B) 18 months
   C) 24 months
   D) 30 months
   E) 36 months

39) **Which of the following is true regarding mental retardation in children?**

A) 25% of children with severe mental retardation have associated behavioral problems

B) Seizures are twice as common in children who have mental retardation than the general population

C) Approximately 25% of patients with cerebral palsy have comorbid mental retardation of some degree

D) The correct term for children less than 6 years old suspected of having mental retardation is *global developmental delay*

E) The prevalence of sleep disorders is proportional to intelligence

40) **Which of the following is true regarding eligibility for "Early Intervention Programs" (EIP)?**

A) Infants diagnosed with a syndrome known to be associated with mental retardation become eligible when developmental delays are identified

B) Infants diagnosed with a syndrome known to be associated with mental retardation become eligible at age 3

C) Infants diagnosed with a syndrome known to be associated with mental retardation become eligible at birth

D) Children diagnosed prior to their 3rd birthday should be referred to EIP when developmental delays are identified

E) Children diagnosed prior to their 3rd birthday should be referred to EIP just prior to entering school

Critical Care

41) All of the following interfere with the accuracy of pulse oximetry *EXCEPT* for:

A) Elevated methemoglobinemia
B) Elevated carboxyhemoglobin
C) Impaired perfusion
D) Hypoglycemia
E) Hypothermia

42) Match the diagnoses on the left with the arterial blood gas results on the right

			pH	PCO_2	Bicarb
1)	Respiratory acidosis	(A)	7.25	24	10
2)	Respiratory alkalosis	(B)	7.62	22	37
3)	Metabolic alkalosis	(C)	7.25	60	38
4)	Metabolic acidosis	(D)	7.01	62	12
5)	Respiratory acidosis (compensated)	(E)	7.52	18	10
6)	Respiratory alkalosis (compensated)	(F)	7.36	20	10
7)	Combined acidosis (metabolic – respiratory)	(G)	7.52	34	37
8)	Combined alkalosis (metabolic – respiratory)	(H)	7.36	65	40

43) Following a near drowning episode under which of the following conditions could a child safely be discharged from the ER and observed at home?

A) Brief seizure
B) Child who required CPR in the field who is now stable with a GCS of 15
C) Child submerged less than one minute who received no CPR in the field
D) Child was stable but now tachypneic
E) Stable child who initially aspirated water

44) Which of following statements regarding *hyperventilation syndrome* is true?

  A) It is synonymous with *panic attack*
  B) It is breathing in excess of metabolic requirements resulting in hypercapnia
  C) The safest treatment in the acute setting is breathing into a paper bag
  D) When anxiety is the cause reassurance of the absence of organic pathology will often resole the problem
  E) The absence of chest pain or fever rules out congestive heart failure and pneumonia

45) You are treating a 12 month old child who is febrile, tachypneic, and moderately hypotensive with scattered petechiae on the trunk and purpuric lesions on the ankles. Until a definitive diagnosis is established which of the following would be the most appropriate treatment?

  A) Referral to child protective services for child abuse and neglect
  B) Assume a diagnosis of Henoch Schönlein purpura and observe overnight
  C) IV Ceftriaxone
  D) IV Vancomycin
  E) IV Vancomycin and Ceftriaxone

46) You are asked to give a talk on polyomavirus hominis (BKV) infection. You note that it infects up to 90% of the general population. Midway through your talk, in addition to realizing your fly is opened and your are wearing different color shoes. Fortunately you did note that BKV is an important cause of late onset graft rejection of the following organ:

  A) Liver
  B) Lung
  C) Heart
  D) Ego
  E) Kidney

Dermatology

47) In the following set of questions, for each numbered word or phrase, choose the lettered heading that is MOST CLOSELY ASSOCIATED with it. Lettered headings may be selected once, more than once, or not at all.

1) Inflammation and black dots
2) Complete areas of smooth hair loss
3) Incomplete patches of hair loss with hair shafts of varying lengths
4) Eyebrows are involved
5) Pediatrician preparing for the Boards

(A) Alopecia neurotica
(B) Alopecia totalis
(C) Trichotillomania
(D) Tinea capitis
(E) Alopecia areata

48) A 15-year-old presents with inflammation and severe tenderness and itching of the lateral toe webs and soles of both feet. There is also a foul odor that often "clears the room". There are fissures noted between the toes as well. His 16-year-old brother has similar symptoms. Which of the following is the most likely diagnosis?

A) Scabies
B) Atopic dermatitis
C) Chemical irritation
D) Hyperhidrosis
E) Tinea pedis

49) The rash MOST associated with fifth disease is:

A) Erythema multiforme
B) Erythema marginatum
C) Erythema nodosum
D) Erythema migrans
E) Erythema infectiosum

50) **Which one of the following is associated with Bacterial sepsis due to *Neisseria meningitidis* secondary to acquired protein C deficiency?**

A) Erythema multiforme
B) Erythema migrans
C) Erythema marginatum
D) Gianotti-Crosti syndrome
E) Pyoderma gangrenosum
F) Purpura fulminans

51) **A 9-year-old child presents with tender erythematous nodules on the lower extremities concentrated on the pretibial area. The nodules are very tender. The MOST likely cause of this rash is:**

A) Playing goalie without goalie pads
B) Tuberculosis
C) Inflammatory bowel disease
D) Coccidioidomycosis
E) Blastomycosis
F) Group A *Strep*

52) **A 3-month-old infant presents with a severe rash concentrated on the face and scalp. The rash is yellow in color and scaly, with patches that are ulcerated and crusting. Some petechiae and purpura are noted as well. The BEST step in managing this problem would be:**

A) Reassurance
B) Zinc supplements
C) Hydrocortisone cream and nystatin ointment
D) Moisturizing lotions and soap
E) Skin biopsy

53) **You are called by the local nurse practitioner who is baffled by a rash in a 4-year-old patient. The nurse describes the rash as flat, non-pruritic papules on the face and extremities, and also notes some lesions on the buttocks, but not the trunk. You, of course, tell her that the diagnosis is:**

A) Psoriasis
B) Atopic dermatitis
C) Erythema multiforme
D) Erythema erythema
E) Gianotti-Crosti syndrome
F) Pityriasis rosea

54) **Treatment of tinea capitis with oral griseofulvin should include:**

A) Lipid-containing foods at the time the medication is given
B) Baseline complete blood count and liver function tests
C) A trial of antifungal shampoo and other agents before using any oral agent
D) Fat-free foods at the time of administration
E) The use of no other medications, especially topical steroids, that will hasten the spread of the infection

55) **A 15-year-old boy has a large number of comedones on his face, but no papules or pustules. Of the following, the treatment of choice for this boy is:**

A) A regimen of face scrubbing with soap and a washcloth
B) The application of mentholated cream as a cleanser
C) The application of retinoic acid cream to his face
D) Oral administration of high doses of vitamin A
E) Oral administration of tetracycline

56) Eczematous changes in association with hypopigmentation are MOST likely a result of:

A) Dietary zinc deficiency
B) Vitamin E deficiency
C) Essential fatty acid deficiency
D) Biotin deficiency
E) Kwashiorkor

Endocrinology

57) A newborn in your practice has a positive result on her newborn screen for hypothyroid. Which of the following is the MOST appropriate *next* step in managing this patient?

A) Obtain a serum Free T4 and hold treatment pending results
B) Obtain a serum Free T4 and begin treatment immediately
C) Obtain a serum TSH and hold treatment pending results
D) Obtain a serum TSH and begin treatment immediately
E) Obtain a total T3 and begin treatment immediately

58) Children who develop hypothyroidism after what which age can expect to have no *permanent impairment* of intellectual or neurological function?

A) 3 months
B) 6 months
C) 12 months
D) 18 months
E) 36 months

59) At which age must hypothyroidism be diagnosed and treated in order to reduce the risk for impaired intellectual function and neuropsychological development?

A) 3 months
B) 6 months
C) 12 months
D) 18 months
E) 36 months

60) The most appropriate treatment for idiopathic central precocious puberty is:

A) FSH
B) LH
C) Leuprolide
D) Growth hormone
E) GnRH

61) You are evaluating a 16 year old boy whose SMR is 2 and whose parents are concerned over his lack of pubertal development and being somewhat shorter than they would expect. His growth was in the 60th percentile until age 12 and has gradually dropped to the 5th percentile. His weight remained in the 50th percentile. The boys bone age is 14. The parents note that his older brother was also a "slow grower" The MOST likely explanation for the findings is:

A) Familial short stature
B) Constitutional growth delay
C) Hypothyroidism
D) Crohn Disease
E) Nutritional deficiency

62) You are evaluating a 16 year old boy who has dropped from the 50th percentile for both weight and height since age 11. He otherwise feels fine. Which of following would be the most appropriate initial step in establishing the underlying cause of the above presentations

A) TSH
B) Free T4
C) T4/TS
D) Erythrocyte sedimentation rate
E) Serum cortisol levels

63) You suspect a growth hormone deficiency as the underlying cause of short stature in a child. The most appropriate initial screen would be to order a:

A) Growth hormone
B) GnRH
C) Tissue transglutaminase antibody
D) IGF-1
E) Erythrocyte sedimentation level

64) You suspect celiac disease to be the underlying cause of a child's short stature. You document a normal IgA concentration. The most appropriate initial screening test would be:

A) Erythrocyte sedimentation rate
B) Small bowel biopsy
C) Stool glutinoid binding mucosal binding protein
D) Tissue transglutaminase antibody level
E) Stool for reducing substances

65) You are evaluating a 17 year old girl who has been complaining of gradually increasing headaches and visual deficits. Despite an SMR of 4 she has not started to menstruate. You order an MRI of the brain the most appropriate study to order would be a serum

A) TSH
B) GnRH
C) LH
D) Prolactin
E) IGF-1:

66) The family of an 8-year-old boy expresses concern about his growth. Past records reveal that the child has been healthy and that height and weight have consistently been at the 5%ile. The father's height is 163 cm (64 inches) and the mother's is 152 cm (60 in). Physical examination reveals a healthy, prepubertal boy. The bone age is 8. Which of the following patterns of growth and sexual maturation is MOST likely in this child?

Adult Stature	Onset	Rate of Progression
A) 3%ile	Normal	Normal
B) 25%ile	Delayed	Slow
C) 50%ile	Early	Rapid
D) 50%ile	Early	Slow
E) 50%ile	Normal	Normal

67) Which of the following is *most frequently* associated with hypoparathyroidism in children?

A) Subcutaneous calcification
B) Mucocutaneous candidiasis
C) Hematuria
D) Hypertension
E) Hypoglycemia

68)   You are evaluating a 2 year old who is walking bow legged, and whose ankles and wrists seem to be enlarged and there are bumps along his rib cage. He is below the 25th percentile for height and weight. CBC and ESR are within normal limits. Parathyroid hormone, 1, 25 Vitamin D, 25, Vitamin D, and calcium levels are all within normal limits. His alkaline phosphatase levels are markedly elevated and serum phosphate levels are well below normal.

The most likely explanation for these findings is

A)   Nutritional neglect
B)   Physical abuse
C)   Vitamin D dependent rickets Type 1
D)   Vitamin D dependent rickets Type 2
E)   Familial hypophosphatemic rickets

69)   You are evaluating a 2 year old African American lactose intolerant child who is walking bow legged, and whose ankles and wrists seem to be enlarged and there are bumps along his rib cage. The CBC and ESR are within normal limits. Vitamin D, 25, Serum Phosphate and Calcium are all low. Alkaline phosphate and PTH are high.

The most likely explanation for these findings is

A)   Vitamin D deficient rickets
B)   Vitamin D dependent rickets Type 1
C)   Vitamin D dependent rickets Type 2
D)   X- Linked familial hypophosphatemia
E)   Hypophosphatasia

70) You are evaluating a 2 year old who is walking bow legged, and whose ankles and wrists seem to be enlarged and there are bumps along his rib cage. CBC and ESR are within normal limits. Parathyroid hormone and alkaline phosphatase are both high. Serum calcium and phophate are low. The serum Vitamin D 1, 25 is very low. A trial of Vitamin D replacement therapy has been unsuccessful.

The most likely diagnosis is

A) Vitamin D deficient rickets
B) Vitamin D dependent rickets Type 1
C) Vitamin D dependent rickets Type 2
D) X-linked familial hypophosphatemia
E) Poor compliance with treatment

71) You are evaluating a 2 year old who is walking bow legged, and whose ankles and wrists seem to be enlarged and there are bumps along his rib cage. CBC and ESR are within normal limits. Parathyroid hormone, alkaline phosphatase and Vitamin D 1, 25 are all high. Serum calcium and phosphate are low.

The most likely diagnosis is:

A) Vitamin D deficient rickets
B) Vitamin D dependent rickets Type 1
C) Vitamin D dependent rickets Type 2
D) X-linked familial hypophosphatemia
E) Osteogenic imperfecta Type 2

72) Each of the following are associated with metabolic syndrome in a 16 year old boy except:

A) Fasting triglycerides greater than 150
B) High density lipoprotein cholesterol great than 40
C) Klood pressure greater than 130/85
D) Fasting glucose greater than 100
E) Previously diagnosed type 2 diabetes melitis

73)   A 17-year-old boy is hospitalized because of severe DKA. The patient is on appropriate insulin regimen as prescribed by the endocrinologist. An appropriate diet has been set up by a nutritionist. You review the old chart and note this is his 5th admission for DKA in the past 5 months. Which of the following is the MOST likely cause of the recurrent DKA?

A)   Inappropriate insulin dosing
B)   Dawn effect
C)   Excessive caloric intake
D)   Somogyi effect
E)   Poor compliance

74)   Which of the following statements is TRUE regarding diabetes in children?

A)   Type 1 diabetes is strictly an autoimmune phenomenon
B)   Type 2 diabetes in children is strictly due to insulin resistance
C)   Type 2 diabetes is seen exclusively in obese children.
D)   The younger the child, the more likely they have Type 2
E)   The younger the child, the more likely they have Type 1

75)   In the following set of questions, decide if each numbered choice applies to (A) only, (B) only, both (C), or neither (D):

1)   "Incidental" diagnosis on routine physical in asymptomatic patient
2)   Vaginal monilial infection can be a presenting sign
3)   Acanthosis nigricans
4)   Presence of autoantibodies
5)   Exacerbated by stress/disease
6)   Arcaneis testus

(A) Frequently occurs with Type 1 diabetes
(B) Frequently occurs with Type 2 diabetes
(C) Both
(D) Neither

76) The 7-year-old daughter of a woman with Type 1 diabetes has had several unexplained hypoglycemic seizures. Prior to this time the child had no prior medical problems. Lab studies reveal that the serum concentration of insulin increases during hypoglycemic episodes. Which of the following would be MOST useful in determining the cause of the hypoglycemic seizures?

A) Serum islet cell antibody titers
B) Serum ketones
C) Plasma C-peptide concentration
D) Plasma glucagon concentration
E) Serum anti-insulin antibody titers

77) In the following set of questions, decide if each numbered choice applies to (A) only, (B) only, both (C), or neither (D):

1) Hyperthyroidism
2) Hypothyroidism
3) Immune system involvement
4) Precancerous lesion

(A) Graves' disease
(B) Hashimoto's disease
(C) Both
(D) Neither

5) Owned a diner on the 70s hit TV show Happy Days
6) Usually asymptomatic at presentation
7) Can be hypothyroid at presentation

ENT

78) **Over-the-counter expectorants for coughs and upper respiratory tract infections generally:**

A) Have a substantial antitussive *and* decongestive effect
B) Clinically decrease the viscosity of mucous secretions
C) Have the same effect as compressed powdered candy
D) Increase the volume of secretions but do not affect the viscosity
E) Have an antitussive effect and should be recommended for bedtime use only

79) **Tonsils usually reach their maximum size in children at what age?**

A) 1 to 1-1/2 years
B) 2 to 3 years
C) 5 to 7 years
D) 10 to 12 years
E) 16 to 18 years

80) **In the following set of questions, for each numbered word or phrase, choose the lettered heading that is MOST CLOSELY ASSOCIATED with it. Lettered headings may be selected once, more than once, or not at all.**

1) Wet inspiratory stridor
2) High-pitched inspiratory stridor
3) Expiratory stridor

(A) Tracheomalacia
(B) Laryngomalacia
(C) Paralyzed vocal cords
(D) Stricken with fear and panic

81) An 18-month-old boy has a bark-like cough and inspiratory stridor. An x-ray study of the soft tissue of the neck shows subglottic narrowing. Based on these clinical and radiological findings, the MOST likely diagnosis is:

A) Bacterial tracheitis
B) Epiglottitis
C) Viral croup
D) Subglottic hemangioma
E) Foreign body aspiration

82) A 12-year-old presents with fever, "hot potato voice," and trismus. He was diagnosed with pharyngitis over one week ago and is not sure if the culture was positive. They took an antibiotic but stopped because it "did not taste good". All of the following is likely in this patient are EXCEPT:

A) Bilateral tonsillar inflammation is the cause of the voice change
B) Penicillin would be the treatment of choice
C) Parenteral antibiotics are needed
D) Beta hemolytic strep could be the cause
E) Anaerobic organisms could be the cause

83) A 2 -year-old boy presents with a history of purulent nasal discharge from the left nostril for one week. Physical examination reveals copious foul-smelling discharge with some edema of the nares. The MOST likely diagnosis is:

A) Unilateral choanal atresia
B) Bacterial sinusitis
C) Allergic rhinitis
D) Juvenile angiofibroma
E) Foreign body

84) **A 5-year-old girl presents with pain behind her ear for 2 days. On physical examination, she has a temperature of 39.8C, and you note swelling over the postauricular area with outward and downward displacement of the pinna. Which of the following is the MOST likely diagnosis?**

A) Mastoiditis
B) Parotiditis
C) Mumps
D) Otitis media with effusion
E) Cholesteatoma

85) **Documentation of which one of the following describes an *absolute* indication for tonsillectomy?**

A) Seven episodes of tonsillitis in a year
B) Tonsillar hypertrophy
C) Peritonsillar abscess
D) Retropharyngeal abscess
E) Obstructive sleep apnea
F) Snoring audible enough to cross state lines

86) **An 8-year-old develops acute onset of bilateral hearing loss confirmed as sensorineural. The MOST likely cause of this problem would be:**

A) Drug toxicity
B) Viral illness
C) Previously undetected bilateral acoustic neuromas
D) Foreign body
E) Autoimmune disease

87)   Tympanometry would be MOST useful when used to:

A) Diagnose otitis media
B) Diagnose otitis externa
C) Identify source of middle ear effusion
D) Identify conductive hearing loss
E) Diagnose impaired mobility of the tympanic membrane

88)   A 3-year-old girl is referred for evaluation of a mass in the midline of the neck. The mass has been present for several months and has not changed size. She has been otherwise well.

On physical exam, you note an alert, well-developed, well-nourished child who is afebrile, height <5%ile, and weight 90%ile. There is a 1.8 cm cystic lesion approximately just above the thyroid cartilage. The thyroid gland cannot be felt. There is no cervical adenopathy. No other significant physical findings are noted. Prior to removal of the mass, which of the following would be MOST appropriate?

A) Needle aspiration of the mass
B) Radionuclide thyroid scan
C) Lateral view x-ray study of the neck
D) Antithyroid antibody titer
E) Determination of the serum thyroglobulin concentration

89)   Which of the following would be the most appropriate antibiotic to use to treat a dental abscess in a 5 year old?

A) Ciprofloxacin
B) Clindamycin
C) Penicillin
D) Augmentin
E) Ceclor

90)   The most appropriate intervention in a 15 month old who is bottle and breast fed and has
       developed dental caries would be to:

A) Discontinue nocturnal breast feeding
B) Continue breastfeeding but have mom take fluoride supplementation
C) Discontinue bottle feeding at night
D) A and C
E) Start vitamins with fluoride

91)   Which of the following is the most common complication of otitis media?

A) Hearing loss
B) Mastoiditis
C) Meningitis
D) Sinusitis
E) Intracranial abscess

92)   A 12 year old presents with several weeks of nasal congestion, along with a persistent cough
       at night that keeps him up. He also has been experiencing malaise, poor appetite,
       intermittent fever and headache. The most likely diagnosis would be:

A) Allergic rhinitis
B) Aseptic meningitis
C) Encephalopathy
D) Chronic sinusitis
E) Acute sinusitis

93) A child presents with bilateral ear pain, a low grade fever, erythematous TM, with good movement with insufflation, distinct landmarks and a peaked curve on tympanometry would suggest which diagnosis and treatment?

A) Otitis media / amoxicillin
B) Otitis media/ amoxicillin – clavulanic acid
C) Otitis externa/ cortisone based ear drops
D) Myringitis/ ibuprofen
E) Viral infection/ no treatment

94) Appropriate antibiotic treatment of conjunctivitis and otitis media would be:

A) Amoxicillin
B) Amoxicillin/ clavulanic acid
C) Gentamicin eyedrops and amoxicillin
D) Antibiotic eardrops and eyedrops
E) Supportive care only

95) You are evaluating a 17 year old female for a sore throat of 5 days duration. Rapid strep and throat culture for Group a beta hemolytic strep was negative. She is sexually active She was treated for a cervical chlamydia infection last month. On physical examination you note red patches of the pharynx, with no exudate and no petechiae.

The most appropriate test to establish a diagnosis would be:

A) Chlamydia throat culture
B) Chlamydia and gonorrhea nucleic acid amplification screening
C) Gonorrhea throat culture
D) Serum monospot
E) No treatment or diagnosing testing

ER

96) **With regards to sexual abuse, which of the following is true?**

A) A normal genito-anal exam all but rules out sexual abuse
B) A crescentic hymen on physical exam is pathognomonic for sexual assault
C) Labial adhesions are most commonly caused by repeated sexual abuse and are best treated with estrogen creams
D) Posterior hymenal tears on vaginal exam are more consistent with sexual abuse
E) Physical exam should focus on the labia majora and minora for signs of abuse

97) **A mom, carrying her 18 month old son, runs into your office leaving skid marks in the waiting room as she comes to a screeching halt. She places her son at your feet just as you are completing your notes on the 300th URI you have seen that hour. She reports hearing a "thud" in the living room where her child was playing and finding him "not breathing, blue and unresponsive".**

Although not CPR trained, she regularly watches *Grey's Anatomy, House, and Scrubs* and knew what to do immediately. She even barked out orders to the neighbor who was "paged stat" to her living room. . . The child immediately came to and is now playing comfortably with the stuffed teletubby on your desk. After you take a more complete history and conduct a physical, your choice of treatment in this case would be:

A) EEG, EKG, and loading dose of Dilantin pending full neurological workup and consultation
B) Observation overnight and 12 lead EKG, EEG, and CT scan if there is any evidence of head trauma
C) Reassurance and a trial of iron supplementation
D) A humble concession that you need to watch *Grey's Anatomy* more often because that show IS damned realistic except for the active social life you don't recall experiencing.
E) Chem 23 panel and arrangement for a Medic Alert bracelet in case there is any recurrence

98) **Which of the following represents the most accurate statement with regards to sexual abuse?**

A) Awkward procedures like pubic hair sampling should never be delayed
B) With a thorough physical exam, physical evidence of abuse is almost always present
C) Overall, transmission of sexually transmitted diseases is a rare occurrence
D) Most cases of sexual abuse are perpetrated by someone unknown to the family
E) STD screening should be done in the ER regardless of risk

99) **Which of the following is the most appropriate location for insertion of an intraosseous needle?**

A) Midpoint of the tibial shaft
B) Midpoint of the femoral shaft, in the midline
C) 1 cm proximal to the tibial tuberosity
D) Anteromedial tibia, 2 cm distal to the tuberosity
E) Mid sternum

100) **Match the diagnoses on the left with the clinical descriptions on the right.**

1) Ureteropelvic junction obstructions
2) Dysmenorrhea
3) Acute intermittent porphyria
4) Psychogenic abdominal pain (conversion disorder)

(A) Labile 13 year old with a depressed parent
(B) Paroxysmal abdominal pain along with headaches, dizziness and syncope
(C) Painless bloody diarrhea
(D) Cramping, dull, midline pain
(E) Recurrent episodes of periumbilical and midepigastric cramps with episodic vomiting

101) Which of the following is the MOST appropriate initial treatment of severe hypertension in a known asthmatic?

A) Benzodiazepines
B) Morphine
C) Cold compresses
D) Vasodilators
E) Beta-blockers

102) An 18 year-old comatose boy is brought to the ER. The friend who accompanied him to the ER states he noticed that the patient took a small fistful of some pills earlier, but knows of no other history. Temperature is 37.2 C, heart rate is 45/min, RR is 6/min, and BP is 75/45 mm Hg. Pupils are 1.0 mm in diameter. There is no nystagmus or spontaneous lacrimation. The patient is responsive only to deep painful stimuli and is hyporeflexic. Ingestion of which of the following substances is MOST likely?

A) Diphenhydramine
B) Tricyclic antidepressants
C) Organophosphates
D) Methylphenidate
E) Opiates

103) You are evaluating an *afebrile* 3-year-old boy who will not bear weight on his legs. Due to inconsistencies in the history, you suspect child abuse. You order x-ray studies of the lower extremities,[2] which show no evidence of any fractures. The MOST appropriate next step in management would be to order:

A) A conventional CT scan of the legs
B) Technetium bone scan
C) Close follow-up for signs of further abuse
D) MRI of the legs
E) PET scan of his pet's legs

---

[2] Known as "legs" to the rest of the world.

104) The reduction of intracranial pressure following the IV administration of mannitol to patients with cerebral edema is caused by decrease in:

A) Cerebral volume
B) Brain water volume
C) CSF volume
D) Cardiac output
E) Respiratory rate

105) A 5-year-old boy was found drowning in the family swimming pool and was resuscitated on-site by EMS. He arrives at the ER in minimal respiratory distress with vital signs stable. As a precaution, he is hospitalized and becomes tachypneic over the next 18 hours.

The initial chest x-ray demonstrated a fine reticular infiltrate. A second x-ray taken later shows evidence of pulmonary edema. Clinically, the oxygen saturations decrease and he requires oxygen, and you note audible crackles. The respiratory distress increases and you intubate and start the child on mechanical ventilation. Which of the following would BEST explain the deteriorating status?

A) Poor initial resuscitation
B) Tension pneumothorax
C) Pulmonary embolism
D) Acute respiratory distress syndrome
E) Aspiration pneumonia

106) A 3-year-old with a history of bloody diarrhea and a high fever is in your waiting room. A frantic pharmaceutical rep (who dropped his box of donuts covered with promotional stickers because the child is having a generalized seizure) calls you out. You step over and onto some of the donuts and realize you must:

A) Ask for new donuts
B) Administer 3% Normal Saline
C) Administer a Normal Saline bolus
D) Treat for *Salmonella* once the seizure is brought under control
E) Treat for *Shigella* once the seizure is brought under control

107) **You would be correct in making a presumptive diagnosis of child abuse in each of the following situations EXCEPT:**

A) A 4-year-old with evenly distributed purpuric lesions on the lower extremities
B) Fracture of the posterior ribs following a fall from a chair
C) A 6-year-old with several fractures in different stages who has otherwise been doing well
D) A 2-year-old hyperactive child with a fracture noted on the sternum of the chest
E) A 6-year-old with a fracture of the scapula
F) A 6-year-old with a spiral fracture on the mid shaft of the humerus

108) **A 6-year-old is brought to the emergency department after being struck by a car driven by a driver talking on a cell phone.[3] He presents with abdominal tenderness, decreased bowel sounds, and some guarding, but no rebound tenderness. Your INITIAL step should be:**

A) Abdominal plain film
B) Abdominal ultrasound
C) Airway assessment
D) Evaluate cap refill while preparing for IV placement and intraosseous line if necessary
E) Computed tomography

109) **Regarding the physical abuse of children which of the following is true?**

A) Minor injuries do not represent a pattern of abuse
B) The age of a bruise can always be determined by the color
C) Bruises from accidental injury can be identified by location.
D) Cultural healing practices that leave skin marks have not been well described
E) Burn marks in a splash pattern are typically a result of deliberate abuse

---

[3] The driver is brought in moments later with "cell phone impaled tympanic membrane syndrome."

110) A 20-year-old student has an injured arm. X-ray study of the distal humerus reveals a fracture in the supracondylar region. Which of the following is the most concerning complication of such an injury?

A) Neurovascular compromise
B) Growth plate injury
C) Fat embolism
D) Pulmonary embolism
E) Hypercalcemia secondary to immobilization

111) One hour ago a 10-year-old boy was a passenger in an automobile that was involved in a collision. The child was wearing a lap belt and did not lose consciousness. He now has abdominal pain but no headache.

The patient is well oriented and alert. Physical exam reveals no evidence of bone fractures. There is mild bruising where the lap belt crossed the abdomen, and the abdomen is tender throughout. Lab studies reveal a HGB of 9.0 g/dL and a HCT of 27%. You suspect that the patient has a ruptured spleen.

Which of the following would be the *most appropriate* next step in confirming the diagnosis?

A) CT of the abdomen with IV contrast
B) US of the abdomen
C) CT of the abdomen without contrast
D) Paracentesis
E) Serial HCT determinations

112) In a household where 50 ore more episodes of domestic violence takes place what percentage of children are likely to be abused by their fathers?

A) 10%
B) 30%
C) 50%
D) 75%
E) 100%

113) **Which of the following statements regarding sports related head injuries is true?**

   A) The majority of concussive injuries in young athletes is now closely monitored and reported
   B) Mouthguard use while preventing dental injury, has no beneficial value in preventing concussive injury
   C) The team trainer is an important liaison for the primary care physician in assuring that appropriate protocol for returning to activity is followed
   D) Assigning the correct grade of concussion is the most crucial step in determining management.
   E) Athletes with one concussive episode are two times as likely to have a second one.

114) **Which of the following would be the most important initial step when assessing a fallen football player with a potential cervical spine injury?**

   A) Remove the helmet
   B) Remove the facemask
   C) Palpate the cervical spine for tenderness
   D) Assess the airway
   E) Assess the mechanism of injury

115) **Which of the following is true regarding ankle injuries?**

   A) Improper shoes and poor training are the most common causes of ankle injury
   B) Fracture the 1st metatarsal is commonly seen with inversion injuries
   C) With a minor injury, with no point tenderness or limping , ankle mobilization can proceed within 18 hours
   D) Rest, ice, compression and elevation is most helpful for 48 hours after the ankle injury
   E) Heat should be applied to the injury initially along with elevation

116) **Which of the following is true regarding fentanyl in conscious sedation ?**

   A) Fentanyl has a longer half-life than morphine
   B) Provides sufficient anxiolysis to be used without other agents
   C) If titrated too rapidly can result in chest wall stiffness
   D) It is indicated for non-painful prolonged distressing procedures
   E) Has no role in conscious sedation in children

117) **Each of the following would be helpful nonpharmacological methods to reduce anxiety during painful procedures performed in children** *except*:

   A) Cartoons
   B) Breathing exercises
   C) Video games
   D) Reassuring comments such as "I'm sorry we have to do this"
   E) Music

118) **90 % of allergic reactions to food are due to each of the following** *except* **for:**

   A) Strawberries
   B) Milk
   C) Eggs
   D) Soy
   E) Fish

119) You are evaluating a previously healthy 4 year old who presents to the emergency department with a 1 day history of paroxysmal coughing and posttussive forceful emesis. He was brought to the ER because of 2 episodes of emesis that were blood streaked. The physical example is unremarkable including the absence of any significant abdominal pain or wheeze , rales or rhonchi.

The most likely explanation for the clinical presentation would be:

A) Inexplicable
B) Acute alcohol intoxication
C) Mallory Weiss Tear
D) Peptic Ulcer disease
E) Gastritis

120) **Each of the following is true regarding cyclic vomiting syndrome *except***

A) Amitriptyline and propranolol are effective during acute episodes
B) Intervals of normal health is typical between episodes
C) 3 or more episodes of recurrent vomiting is part of the diagnosis
D) No lab results to support an alternative diagnosis
E) No radiographic evidence to support an alternative diagnosis

Fluids & Lytes

121) **The molar ratio of glucose to sodium in standard oral rehydration solution should not exceed:**

A) 3:1
B) 2:1
C) 1:1
D) 1:2
E) 1:3
F) Molar? This isn't the dental boards! C'mon

122) An 8 week old boy is brought to you in the ER by a panic stricken mother after he has had a generalized seizure. He has had some pretty bad diarrhea according to the mother. You find out that besides breast milk, the *grandmother* has done what she has always done in such cases and gave the baby lots of diluted tea. You order Lytes superstat and are shocked and horrified to find a serum sodium of 110. Your next step is to:

A) Find out more about the tea that packs that kind of punch
B) Order NS 20 cc/KG over 15 – 20 minutes, repeated until clinically warranted
C) Order NS IV maintenance, half over the next 8 hours and the other half over 16 hours
D) Order a 3% saline solution bolus 5 – 6 ml/kg over a few minutes
E) Order a 0.3% saline solution bolus 5 – 6 ml/kg over a few minutes

123) You are caring for an infant diagnosed with hypernatremic dehydration. It is December and you have been a PGY1 for close to 6 months now. You have seen one, done one, taught one, 300 times now, but who is counting. The chief Resident, along with the rest of the residents, decides to go to the Christmas party and you are left to fend for yourself. This child is in good hands because you know that he is at risk for developing a seizure due to :

A) Central pontine myelinolysis
B) The shifting of extra cellular and interstitial fluids
C) Rapid change in sodium concentration
D) Rapid change in glucose concentration
E) Rapid change in the blood ethanol alcohol of the rest of the house staff attending the party

124) A 6-month-old infant presents with a 3-day history of vomiting and diarrhea. You are told that she has been given tap water on demand. Her lab findings include a Na^+ of 115 mEq/L, Cl^- of 80 mEq/L, and serum glucose of 80 mg/dL. While in the waiting area she has a generalized seizure. The MOST appropriate next step is to administer:

A) IV phenytoin
B) Endotracheal intubation
C) Normal saline 20 cc/kg over 20 minutes
D) D_5 0.45% normal saline 10 cc/kg over 20 minutes
E) 3% sodium chloride

125) A 2-year-old has had vomiting, diarrhea, and fever for 5 days. His mother has been feeding him a homemade mixture of sugar, salt, and water. Which of the following is the most likely cause of the seizure?

A) Cerebral edema
B) Bacterial meningitis
C) Fever
D) Hypokalemia
E) Hypocalcemia

126) An 18-month-old has a one-week history of vomiting and diarrhea. His grandmother has given him a rice, water, and salt mixture. He appears lethargic and irritable and has doughy abdominal skin.[4] Which of the following lab results would BEST explain the findings?

A) Serum chloride concentration of 97 mEq/L
B) Blood glucose concentration of 95 mg/dL
C) Blood glucose concentration of 170 mg/dL
D) Serum sodium concentration of 125 mEq/L
E) Serum sodium concentration of 165 mEq/L

127) Each of the following is associated with hemolytic uremic syndrome (HUS) EXCEPT for :

A) Hyponatremia
B) Hypokalemia
C) Metabolic acidosis
D) Hyperphosphatemia
E) Consumptive thrombocytopenia

---

[4] Not unlike the doughy abdominal skin of the average male studying for the boards.

128) A child with asthma is examined during an episode that has lasted for a few hours. Except for tachypnea, wheezing, and retractions, there are no abnormal findings on physical examination.

ABG reveals a pH of 7.25, PCO2 of 30, and PO2 of 70. The probable cause of the acidemia is:

A) Respiratory owing to CO2 retention
B) Metabolic owing to renal compensation
C) Metabolic owing to reduced cardiac output
D) Respiratory owing to excessive CO2 loss
E) Metabolic owing to poor tissue oxygenation

129) In the face of hypernatremia in order to maintain homeostasis, idiogenic osmoles are produced in which of the following tissue:

A) Testicular
B) Renal
C) Spleen
D) Central Nervous System
E) Both A and D

130) Which of the following is a true statement regarding electrolytes and osmotic gradients?

A) Hypernatremia is always synonymous with hyperosmolality
B) Hyponatremia is always synonymous with hypoosmolality
C) Ethanol and methanol do not contribute to serum osmolality
D) The presence of ethanol and methanol leads to the movement of fluid across cell membranes
E) When BUN is *chronically elevated* urea contributes to effective osmolality

131) Which of the following would be commonly seen in Cushing Syndrome?

A) Edema
B) Hypertension
C) Decreased body weight
D) Hypernatremia
E) Hyponatremia

132) Each of the following would cause a respiratory alkalosis *except* for:

A) Pneumonia
B) Asthma
C) Salicylate toxicity
D) Barbiturate toxicity
E) Pulmonary edema

133) Each of the following are considered causes of respiratory acidosis except for:

A) Spinal cord injury
B) Myasthenia crisis
C) Guillain-Barré syndrome
D) Nicotine toxicity
E) Botulism

134) Each of the following is an adverse consequences of severe acidemia *except:*

A) Hyperventilation
B) Dyspnea
C) Arteriole dilation
D) Enhanced cardiac contractility
E) Insulin resistance

135) Each of the following are considered causes of metabolic acidosis with a normal anion gap except for:

A) Diarrhea
B) Pancreatic fistula
C) Hypoaldosteronism
D) Ethylene glycol ingestion
E) Renal tubular acidosis.

Genetics

136) **Each of the following is true regarding Down syndrome (Trisomy 21) EXCEPT:**

A) The risk for transmission is higher if the mother is the carrier of a balanced translocation
B) Children with Down syndrome due to a parental translocation are phenotypically different from those due to standard trisomy
C) Mothers in their 20s have more children with Down syndrome than any other age group
D) If the mother has a translocation, the risk of recurrence is 14%
E) In the absence of translocation, the risk of recurrence is 1%

137) **Glucose G6PD deficiency occurring in a female patient could best be explained by:**

A) It can't be explained
B) Klinefelter's syndrome
C) Noonan's syndrome
D) Fanconi anemia
E) Complete androgen insensitivity syndrome

138) **An 8-year-old boy diagnosed with mental retardation is sent for genetic studies. DNA analysis reveals an expanded segment of the CGG segment of DNA in the q27 region of the X chromosome. Which of the following will most likely be found in this patient at puberty?**

A) An accelerated growth spurt
B) Macroorchidism
C) Breast enlargement
D) Further deterioration of intellect
E) Progressive myopathy

139) You are called upon by a couple who have 2 children with Lesch-Nyhan syndrome and a 12-year-old boy who is unaffected by the disease. The parents call you at 3AM because they can't sleep and to find out the chances of their 12-year-old son having an affected child of his own when he starts a family in the distant future.

Now you can't sleep either. You turn on your night light, remove the crust from your eyes, and tell them:

Since Lesch-Nyhan syndrome is inherited in an X-linked recessive manner, you fall back to sleep while the parents are speaking with you and they wake you up and you then tell them that the risk that any child of an unaffected brother male will be affected is:

A) No greater than that of any person in the general population regardless of gender.
B) 25% regardless of gender
C) 50% if the child is a girl and 0% if the child is a boy.
D) 50% if the child is a boy and 0% if the child is a girl.
E) >99% regardless of the gender.
F) Much lower if they had been considerate enough to call you during regular office hours

140) Each of the following is associated with Cri-du – Chat syndrome EXCEPT:

A) Macrocephaly
B) Epicanthal folds
C) Cardiac defects
D) Cat like cry
E) Psychomotor retardation

141) Each of the following are associated with Russel Silver syndrome EXCEPT

A) Cardiac defects
B) Abnormalities in the 5th finger
C) Triangle face
D) Wide spaced teeth
E) Normal head circumference

142) You are evaluating an infant with a hairy back. Long curly eyebrows, long philtrum, wide spaced teeth, hearing loss and a small head. The most likely diagnosis is:

A) Rubinstein Taybi Syndrome
B) Russel Silver Syndrome
C) Cornelia de Lange Syndrome
D) Contestant on American Idol
E) Noonan syndrome

143) You are evaluating a child with macroglossia, hemihypertrophy, cardiomegaly, and hepatomegaly. The most likely diagnosis is:

A) Wilms tumor
B) Noonan Syndrome
C) Russel Silver Syndrome
D) Rubinstein Taybi Syndrome
E) Beckwith Wiedemann Syndrome

144) You are evaluating a patient with broad thumbs and great toes, as well as a beaked nose, and cardiac abnormalities

The most likely diagnosis is:

A) Noonan syndrome
B) Russel Silver Syndrome
C) Rubinstein Taybi Syndrome
D) Beckwith Wiedemann Syndrome.
E) Pierre Robin Syndrome

145)   Each of the following are associated with Klinefelter syndrome EXCEPT:

   A)   Increased risk for breast cancer
   B)   Testosterone replacement therapy
   C)   XYY Karyotype
   D)   Intellectual ability *slightly* below the general population
   E)   Leading cause of male infertility

146)   Which of the following medications are considered to be safe during pregnancy?

   A)   Warfarin
   B)   Heparin
   C)   ACE inhibitors
   D)   Valproic Acid
   E)   Carbamazepine

147)   You are evaluating a newborn who has deviation of the nose to one side, feet that remain medially rotated, and the right outer ear folded down.

   The most likely explanation would be:

   A)   Gestational diabetes
   B)   Eclampsia
   C)   Anticonvulsant exposure
   D)   Oligohydramnios
   E)   Fetal alcohol syndrome

148) A boy in your practice is born with a tracheoesophageal fistula (TEF) with no other abnormal physical findings. The parents are concerned about the possibility of conceiving a child with the same problem. The correct answer would be:

A) Boys have a 50% chance of being born with a TEF
B) The chances that it would occur in the general population
C) 25% regardless of gender
D) 4% risk of recurrence regardless of gender
E) 4% risk for boys only

149) You are evaluating an infant born with a persistent patent ductus arteriosis and documented fetal anuria.

Exposure to which of the following medications would BEST explain this combination of findings.

A) Serotonin reuptake inhibitors
B) Heparin
C) Acetaminophen
D) Amoxicillin
E) ACE inhibitors

150) Exposure to which of the following best explains an infant born with an atrial septal defect and thyroid disturbances.

A) ACE inhibitors
B) Heparin
C) Serotonin reuptake inhibitors
D) Lithium
E) Acetaminophen

GI

151) **Which one of the following can be a contributing factor to chronic non-specific diarrhea in the toddler?**

A) High-fat diet
B) Reduced fecal bile acids
C) Juices with equal concentrations of fructose and glucose
D) 2% milk
E) Restricted fluid intake

152) **Treatment of chronic non-specific diarrhea would include:**

A) Reduction of dietary fiber
B) Cholestyramine and bismuth subsalicylate
C) Increase of daily fluid intake
D) Replacement of grape and orange juice with apple and pear juice
E) Reduction of fat intake by half

153) **Which of the following is *MOST* true about recurrent abdominal pain (RAP)?**

A) It is more common in super achieving children than in those under less pressure
B) Onset in a child older than 4 years of age would require a more aggressive search for a structural abnormality as the cause
C) A history of previous appendectomy and/or migraines is common
D) School absenteeism is common and, given the intensity of pain, private home tutoring is the best option
E) Recurrent abdominal pain is a "diagnosis of exclusion".

154) Match each number (GI disorder) to its corresponding diagnostic test on the right.

1) Presence of chronic inflammation
2) Pernicious anemia
3) Carbohydrate absorption
4) Integrity of intestinal lymphatic system

(A) D-xylose absorption study
(B) Elevated ESR
(C) CBC
(D) Stool pH

155) An 18-hour-old infant has bilious stained emesis following 3 initial feedings. The prenatal and delivery history are unremarkable. On physical exam, the infant is quiet. The occasional peristaltic waves are noted and the abdomen is not distended. Which of the following findings is MOST likely on further radiologic evaluation of this infant?

A) GE reflux
B) Pyloric hypertrophy
C) A "double bubble" sign
D) Malrotation
E) A choledochal duct cyst

156) Which of the following can be seen with "irritable bowel syndrome"?

A) Persistent vomiting
B) Recurrent diarrhea
C) Short stature
D) The absence of pain
E) Hematochezia

157) A 3-year-old boy presents to you with a sudden onset of paroxysmal, colicky pain that started 6 hours ago. The pain comes and goes. He is and has otherwise been healthy. On physical examination there is right upper quadrant tenderness, rectal exam is normal, and stools are guaiac negative. You suspect a diagnosis of intussusception. Each of the following is true regarding intussusception EXCEPT:

A) A guaiac negative stool can be a result of this being an early presentation
B) After reduction via air contrast enema, 90% of the time there will be no recurrence
C) You would expect to find a sausage-like mass on the left lower quadrant
D) It is the most common cause of intestinal obstruction in children of age 3 months to 6 years.
E) Bilious vomiting can develop

158) Which of the following is associated with ariboflavinosis?

A) Cheilosis
B) Xerophthalmia
C) Aphonia
D) Glossitis
E) Oxaluria

159) A 3-year-old boy presents with recurrrent diarrhea. The child had pneumococcal pneumonia at 1 year of age, and meningitis developed at 2 years of age. IV IgG therapy was initiated 6 months ago. Lab studies show that serum IgG, IgA, and IgM concentrations are decreased. CBC and differential are normal. Which of the following is the MOST likely etiology of the recurrent diarrhea?

A) Lactase deficiency
B) Rotavirus infection
C) *Giardia lamblia* infection
D) *Entamoeba histolytica* infection
E) Enterovirus infection

160) One could expect to see low serum albumin levels with each of the following conditions EXCEPT:

A) Kwashiorkor
B) Ascites
C) Inflammatory bowel disease
D) Nephrotic syndrome
E) Hepatitis A

161) A 17-year-old varsity quarterback in your practice is at your office for a school physical in early September. He is being pursued by several universities to play football.[5] The football team has already been training since August 8th. With the exception of his being noticeably icteric, his physical examination is benign. Additional history, laboratory, and physical findings are MOST likely to reveal

A) History of alcohol abuse and severe dehydration
B) Similar past history in the patient as well as his male siblings[6] with elevated unconjugated bilirubin levels and otherwise normal lab findings
C) Low hematocrit on CBC with the elevated bilirubin due to hemolysis secondary to low grade crush injuries while getting tackled
D) Evidence of acute hepatitis A due to the high risk of the team drinking from the same bottles of sports drinks
E) Evidence of undetected chronic hepatitis

162) Each of the following is an increased risk factor for developing hemolytic uremic syndrome after a child is infected with the causative enterohemorrhagic *E. coli* EXCEPT:

A) Older age
B) Use of antimotility medication
C) Use of antibiotics
D) Elevated WBC
E) Presence of prolonged diarrhea

---

[5] And enroll in the gluteus maximus–olecranon process comparative analysis major.
[6] Also known as brothers to the lay public, by the way.

163) A 12-year-old boy was recently treated with amoxicillin for 10 days for group *Streptococcus* pharyngitis. One week after amoxicillin is discontinued, severe diarrhea develops. The MOST likely cause of this problem is:

A) Norwalk viral infection
B) Shigella infection
C) Toxin-induced colitis
D) Immune reaction to antibiotics
E) Ulcerative colitis

164) Each of the following is true regarding Alpha 1 –antitrypsin deficiency *except* for:

A) It is the most common genetic cause of acute liver disease in children
B) It is the most common genetic cause of chronic liver disease in children
C) It is the most common genetically caused disorder necessitating liver transplantation in children
D) Markedly elevated transaminase values are seen in toddlers
E) It can present as neonatal hepatitis syndrome in children

165) Which of the following would be the most appropriate management of a 3 month old infant who is spitting up after feedings but is otherwise asymptomatic. The weight and height are at ht 60th percentile. Which of the following would be appropriate treatment?

A) Change to hypoallergenic formula
B) Thicken formula with rice cereal
C) Put the infant to sleep in the prone position
D) Reassure the mother
E) Start omeprazole

166) **Which one of the following is typical of acute gastroenteritis secondary to rotavirus?**

A) Bilious vomiting
B) Occurrence during the summer
C) Bloody diarrhea
D) The absence of respiratory symptoms
E) Non-bilious vomiting

167) **Each of the following are true statements regarding the most recently licensed vaccine for rotavirus** *except:*

A) It is a live vaccine
B) It has been associated with intussusception
C) It should be administered at 2,4 and 6 months of age
D) The 3rd dose should not be given later than 32 weeks of age
E) The 1st dose should be given between 6 and 12 weeks of age

GU

168) **Each of the following can be explained by an alternative etiology other than sexual abuse in a pre-adolescent girl *EXCEPT* for:**

A) Malodorous vaginal discharge
B) Anterior hymenal tears
C) Condylomata vaginitis
D) Vaginal chlamydia trachomatis infection
E) Bacterial vaginosis

169) A 3-year-old boy has swelling, erythema, and a firm tender area in the left scrotum. The right testis is palpable and appears normal. Which of the following is the MOST likely diagnosis?

A) Epididymitis
B) Hydrocele
C) Inguinal hernia
D) Torsion of the appendix testes
E) Varicocele

170) A 4-year-old girl was toilet trained approximately one year ago. She has developed diurnal enuresis noted by her daycare director. The physical examination is normal, and there is nothing stressful in the child's life to precipitate this problem. Which of the following is the MOST appropriate next step?

A) Imipramine therapy
B) MRI of the lumbosacral spine
C) DDAVP therapy when sleeping outside the home
D) Urinalysis
E) Evaluation under anesthesia for ectopic uretal orifice

171) You are evaluating a 2 month old boy who has bilateral scrotal swelling which is completely non tender. Both sides transilluminate. The most likely diagnosis is:

A) Epididymitis
B) Bilateral inguinal hernia
C) Variocele
D) Hydrocele
E) Torsion of the testicle

172) A 6-year-old girl presents with mild bloody vaginal discharge. The discharge has become has become increasingly malodorous during the past few days. On physical examination, there is no evidence of trauma. Which of the following is the MOST likely cause of the discharge?

A) Hemolytic *Streptococcal* infection
B) Candidal vaginitis
C) Coagulase-positive *Staphylococcal* infection
D) Chlamydia vaginitis
E) Foreign body

173) In which of the following can acute scrotal pain and swelling be seen?

A) Rocky Mountain Spotted Fever
B) Henpecked Shoreline purpura
C) Henoch Schönlein Purpura
D) Intussusception
E) Mycoplasma pneumonia

Heme One

174) Each of the following are vitamin K dependent clotting factors *EXCEPT* for:

A) 2
B) 7
C) 8
D) 9
E) 10

175) Each of the following are associated with a poor prognosis in acute lymphocytic leukemia *EXCEPT* for:

   A) High white blood cell count
   B) Male gender
   C) Pre-B cell
   D) Young age at diagnosis
   E) Slow response to treatment

176) The parents of a child who had unilateral retinoblastoma would like to know the odds of any subsequent children also having the disorder. You correctly tell them:

   A) 5%
   B) 25%
   C) 50%
   D) 75%
   E) 100%

177) You are giving a talk on sickle cell disease to the residents. You need to discuss management and association of sickle cell disease and *stroke*. Each of the following from your handout is correct *EXCEPT* for:

   A) Exchange transfusion can reduce the incidence of stroke
   B) Subtle neuropsychological deficits often result from focal strokes
   C) 6% of children with sickle cell disease develop strokes
   D) CVA's with sickle cell disease is due to both small and large vessel injury
   E) The most accurate diagnostic assessment can be obtained through head CT

178) **Neutrophils are most critical to/or patients who are neutropenic are most vulnerable to:**

A) Opportunistic infections
B) Fungal infections
C) Respiratory tract flora
D) Skin and GI flora
E) Parasitic infections

179) **Which of the following would be the most likely explanation for neutropenia in a patient in your practice?**

A) Poor nutrition
B) Neutered neutropenia
C) Acute lymphocytic leukemia
D) Viral syndrome
E) Cyclic neutropenia

180) **Match the type of anemia on the left to the lab profile on the right. :**

		RDW	Ferritin	FEP	TIBC
1)	Anemia of chronic illness	(A) Elevated	Low	Elevated	Elevated
2)	Beta thalassemia	(B) Low	Normal	Normal	Normal
3)	Iron deficiency	(C) Normal	Normal or High	Elevated	Elevated
4)	Lead poisoning	(D) Decreased	Normal	Elevated	Decreased

181) **In the following set of questions, decide if each numbered choice applies to (A) only, (B) only, both (C), or neither (D):**

1) X-linked recessive
2) Autosomal dominant
3) Heinz bodies
4) Howell-Jolly bodies
5) Aplastic crisis
6) Autosomal recessive

(A) G 6PD deficiency
(B) Hereditary spherocytosis
(C) Both
(D) Neither

182) **In the following set of questions, decide if each numbered choice applies to (A) only, (B) only, both (C), or neither (D):**

1) Thrombocytopenia
2) Increased PTT
3) Abnormal platelet function
4) Eczema
5) Recent viral illness
6) At risk for developing malignancies

(A) Wiskott Aldrich syndrome
(B) Idiopathic thrombocytopenic purpura
(C) Both
(D) Neither

183) **In the following set of questions, decide if each numbered choice applies to (A) only, (B) only, both (C), or neither (D):**

1) Joint pain
2) Bone pain
3) Morning stiffness
4) Lymphadenopathy / hepatosplenomegaly
5) Associated with exposure to microwave towers

(A) JRA
(B) Acute leukemia
(C) Both
(D) Neither

184) An otherwise healthy 12-day-old girl presents with bloody stools. She was born at home and has been exclusively breast-fed. A physician has not yet examined her until now. In addition to a rapid heart rate, you note some blue areas of discoloration on the limbs and buttocks. The rest of the physical exam is unremarkable. The MOST likely diagnosis is:

A) Child abuse
B) Henoch Schönlein purpura
C) Anal fissure
D) Hemorrhagic disease of the newborn
E) Von Willebrand disease

185) Each of the following are associated with Fanconi's anemia EXCEPT:

A) Autosomal recessive inheritance pattern
B) Abnormal skin pigmentation
C) Pancytopenia noted during the first year
D) Renal abnormalities
E) Skeletal abnormalities

186) A 2-1/2-year-old is noted to have Horner's syndrome on the right side. A chest x-ray is ordered and a mass in the upper portion of the mediastinum is noted. The MOST likely diagnosis would be:

A) Lymphoma
B) Tuberculosis
C) Acute lymphocytic leukemia
D) Neuroblastoma
E) Wilms' tumor

187) Regarding iron deficiency anemia, all of the following are true EXCEPT:

A) Serum ferritin levels are lowered
B) Serum iron binding capacity is reduced
C) Serum iron levels are reduced
D) Mean corpuscle volume (MCV) is reduced
E) Iron supplementation is the treatment of choice

188) The "cycles" of cyclic neutropenia consist of periods where neutrophil counts go from normal to neutropenic values. The period of time of "normal values: neutropenic values" is closest to:

A) 1 week normal values: 1 week neutropenic
B) 3 weeks normal values: 1 week neutropenic
C) 8 weeks normal values: 2 weeks neutropenic
D) 16 weeks normal values: 8 weeks neutropenic
E) 20 weeks normal values: 3 weeks neutropenic
F) 22 light years normal values: 2 hours neutropenic

189) Each of the following are associated with the *typical* anemia seen in hemolytic uremic syndrome EXCEPT:

A) Schistocytes
B) Aaron Burr cells
C) Helmet cells
D) Thrombocytopenia
E) Coombs-positive

190) A 4-month-old black infant who has been fed only formula appears pale. Another physician has recently prescribed him iron therapy. HCT is 26% and reticulocyte count 12%; blood smear shows normocytic RBCs and some poikilocytosis and target cells. To manage this infant MOST appropriately you would:

A) Continue iron therapy only
B) Continue the iron therapy and add folic acid supplements
C) Order hemoglobin electrophoresis
D) Discontinue the iron therapy and give folic acid supplements
E) Order examination of the bone marrow

191) Each of the following would be a possible indication for a red blood cell transfusion in a patient with hereditary spherocytosis *except:*

A) Hematocrit lower than 24
B) Severe chronic fatigue
C) Hypersplenism
D) Growth retardation
E) Extramedullary hematopiesis

192) Which of the following lab studies would be *most helpful* in differentiating hereditary spherocytosis from other forms of hemolytic anemia?

A) Haptoglobin levels
B) Unconjugated bilirubin levels
C) Lactic dehydrogenase levels
D) Presence of spherocytes on peripheral smear
E) Direct Coombs

193) **Each of the following is true regarding gallbladder disease in patients with hereditary spherocytosis** *except:*

A) Gallbladder ultrasound is indicated only if symptoms of cholecystitis present
B) Gallbladder ultrasound is indicated every few years after age 10
C) Cholecystectomy is indicated if gallstones are discovered on ultrasound
D) Cholecystectomy is indicated for painful, symptomatic gallstones or bile duct obstruction
E) Cholecystectomy is done electively if splenectomy is indicated

194) **Which of the following is true regarding the risk of cardiotoxicity in patients receiving treatment with** *anthracycline?*

A) Males and females are at equal risk
B) Cardiotoxicity does not occur at relatively low doses
C) Age of diagnosis is not a factor
D) Screening is done every 5 years regardless of cumulative dose
E) Screening is done every 1-5 years depending on cumulative dose

195) **Secondary malignancies are particularly common following:**

A) Non-Hodgkin's lymphoma
B) Hodgkin's Lymphoma
C) Retinoblastoma
D) Neuroblastoma
E) Acute lymphocytic leukemia

196) A 4 year old boy of Mediterranean descent recently treated with an unknown antibiotic for a febrile illness presents with acute onset of pallor. He has not traveled outside the US recently. On physical exam you confirm the pallor and note that the boy is icteric. Abdominal exam is benign, there is no hepatosplenomegaly. The heart rate is 155. WBC is 12.5, hematocrit is 20.

The most likely explanation for the boy's presentation is:

A) Anaphylactic reaction to the antibiotic
B) Hepatitis A.
C) Hereditary spherocytosis
D) Acute lymphoblastic leukemia
E) G6PD deficiency

197) You are evaluating a 2 year old with a painless abdominal mass noted by the mother while dressing her. The child is otherwise completely asymptomatic. Which of the following is the most likely diagnosis?

A) Wilms tumor
B) Neuroblastoma
C) Hepatoblastoma
D) Toxic megacolon
E) Mesenteric adenitis

198) You are evaluating a 2 year old with fever, irritability, and mild periorbital ecchymoses. On physical examination you note a painless abdominal mass. Which of the following is the most likely diagnosis?

A) Wilms tumor
B) Neuroblastoma
C) Retinoblastoma
D) Acute leukemia
E) Child abuse

199) **Each of the following would be considered triggers for a blood transfusion in the absence of physiological compensation *except* for:**

   A) Estimated traumatic blood loss of 25%
   B) Estimated surgical blood loss of 15%
   C) Hematocrit level below 20
   D) Hemoglobin level below 10
   E) A and B

ID

200) **A 2 year old child presents to your office with a history of fever spikes of 104 degrees with cough, coryza, and conjunctivitis. You brilliantly diagnose measles — something that still occurs, mostly on the boards. Which of the following is correct with regards to measles?**

   A) Elevated measles specific IgM at presentation is diagnostic
   B) Good hand washing prevents spread of disease
   C) Patients are contagious from 2 days before becoming symptomatic until 4 days after the onset of the rash
   D) No need to know anything about this measly disease since there is a vaccine
   E) Acute encephalitis is a common complication

201) **During an outbreak of measles, vaccination would be indicated for each of the following *EXCEPT* for:**

   A) A unimmunized 3 year old exposed 2 days earlier
   B) An unimmunized 12 month old exposed 2 days earlier
   C) A symptomatic HIV patient
   D) A 5 year old, who is HIV positive with high CD4 T lymphocyte count, exposed 24 hours earlier
   E) A pregnant woman exposed 2 days ago

202) **All of the following are true about rubella *EXCEPT*:**

A) It is an illness with high morbidity that presents with high fever and an erythematous rash
B) The erythematous rash begins on the face and upper trunk
C) During the pre-vaccine era, inapparent infection was common
D) The period of communicability begins 2 days before the appearance of the rash and lasts another 7 days
E) Infants with congenital rubella should be considered contagious until they are 1 year old or get a confirmed negative by repeat culture
F) Children with rubella are considered contagious for 1 year or the beginning of Oktoberfest, whichever occurs first

203) **Which of the following is a *TRUE* statement about pertussis in infants?**

A) They are most contagious during the catarrhal stage
B) Erythromycin is most effective if given during the catarrhal stage
C) Most cases of pertussis occur among infants who have not yet received a complete course of immunizations .
D) Erythromycin is most effective if given during the paroxysmal stage
E) Maternal antibodies cross the placenta

204) **Confirmed cases of tuberculosis are treated with which one of the following?**

A) Ethambutol
B) Pyrazinamide
C) Rifampin
D) Isoniazid
E) B, C, and D

205) **You have a child in your practice that is at high risk for TB and you suspect that he has it, yet his skin test is negative. You remember that false negatives can occur in each of the following EXCEPT when:**

A) The child has not developed sensitivity yet, but is infected
B) Recent viral infections
C) Poor technique was used
D) Kwashiorkor coexists
E) The child received prior vaccination with BCG

206) **Which of the following is true regarding catch scratch disease (CDS)?**

A) Bacillary angiomatosis is commonly seen in immunocompetent patients with CSD
B) Bacillary peliosis is commonly seen in immunocompetent patients with CSD
C) Both bacillary peliosis and bacillary angiomatosis are commonly seen in patients with CSD
D) The best prevention for CSD is elimination of fleas
E) Removal of cats from the home is important for preventing future disease

207) **A 6-year-old boy was playing with her cat yesterday when she was bitten on the middle finger of her left hand. The parents cleaned the wound thoroughly with soap, water, and hydrogen peroxide, and within several minutes, the finger became sore, swollen, and erythematous. The pain, swelling, and erythema have all increased. Physical examination reveals a temperature of 37.0 C. The most appropriate initial management would be:**

A) Serum antibody for *Bartonella henselae*
B) Blood culture
C) Culture of the wound and obtain a CBC
D) Rabies prophylaxis
E) Download the Cat Scratch Fever Mp3 and sing along.

208) The *most appropriate* treatment for this infection would be:

A) Observation and conservative management
B) Intravenous cefazolin
C) Oral amoxicillin/clavulanic acid
D) Oral penicillin
E) IV penicillin

209) Of the following, the *most specific* diagnostic test for acute herpes simplex virus infection is:

A) An enzyme immunoassay
B) Isolation of the virus by a culture
C) Identification of giant multinucleated cells on a Tzanck smear
D) The development of specific neutralizing antibodies
E) Serum IgM

210) A 6-year-old girl has had varicella for four days. Several of the lesions on her abdomen have developed honey-colored crusts, purulent exudate, and surrounding cellulitis. Gram stain reveals gram-positive cocci in clusters. Which of the following is the MOST appropriate initial treatment?

A) Cefazolin
B) Trimethoprim with sulfamethoxazole
C) Tetracycline
D) Acyclovir
E) Rifampin

211) A 1-month-old infant presents with irritability and poor feeding. Temperature is 40 C. On physical examination you note that the infant is responsive but markedly irritable, with a left tympanic membrane that is bulging and erythematous. The right tympanic membrane is clear. After obtaining the appropriate lab studies, the MOST appropriate antibiotic treatment would consist of:

A) Ampicillin
B) Cefoxitin
C) Cefotaxime
D) Oral amoxicillin with close followup
E) Ampicillin and gentamicin

212) A 4-year-old girl with a 4-day history of fever is admitted to your service. She has had bloody diarrhea for over a week coupled with decreased urinary output.

On physical examination, you note that she is pale and has some edema. CBC is remarkable for a low hematocrit and platelet count. The WBC is normal. Fragmented red cells are noted on the peripheral smear. Urinalysis is positive for blood and the BUN is 75 with a creatinine of 2.9. Your admitting diagnosis is:

A) *Salmonella* diarrhea and sepsis
B) Henoch-Schönlein purpura
C) Shigella
D) Toxic shock syndrome
E) Hemolytic uremic syndrome

213) A 10-week-old infant presents with a 3-day history of a staccato cough. The infant is in mild respiratory distress and is afebrile with stable vital signs.

A CBC reveals a WBC of 12.5 with 22% polys, 5% bands, 65% lymphocytes, and 7% eosinophils. Chest x-ray shows no focal infiltrates, but is remarkable for *diffuse* infiltrates with some hyperinflation. You'd be correct in treating with:

A) IV cefuroxime
B) PO erythromycin
C) Albuterol nebulized treatments
D) High dose corticosteroids
E) Observation

214) A 6-month-old child is diagnosed with pertussis. Each of the following is true regarding azithromycin prophylaxis EXCEPT:

A) It would be indicated for the infant's father
B) It would be indicated for the infant's 3-year-old sibling only if he did not receive his pre-kindergarten booster
C) It would be indicated for the infant's 5-year-old sibling regardless of immunization status
D) It would be indicated in the infant's caretaker at the childcare center
E) It would be indicated for the grandmother living with the family

215) Because of your resonating and charming deep voice, you are asked by the local radio station to render some sound bites in regard to a recent hepatitis A outbreak. You would be MOST correct in suggesting which of the following?

A) Hepatitis A vaccine for all household and sexual contacts within 3 weeks of exposure
B) Immune globulin for all household and sexual contacts within 3 weeks of exposure
C) Immune globulin for all household contacts within 2 weeks of exposure
D) Hepatitis A vaccine for all newborns of mothers with hepatitis A
E) Serological testing of all contacts

216) Which of the following antibiotics should be avoided in patients with known neuromuscular disease?

A) Ampicillin
B) Gentamicin
C) Metronidazole
D) Ceftriaxone
E) Vancomycin
F) None of the above

217) A 10-year-old child weighing more than 11 kg in your practice with a known seizure disorder will be traveling to a part of Africa where there is a risk of exposure to *Plasmodium falciparum.* The parents have already been seen by their internist and have been prescribed prophylactic medications, but the internist rightfully advised them to bring their son to you for management. The BEST way to minimize the risk of contracting malaria secondary to P *falciparum* in this child would be:

A) Primaquine phosphate once a week starting 1 -week prior to the trip and ending 4 weeks after returning
B) Chloroquine once a week during the trip and for 4 weeks upon returning
C) Quinine dihydrochloride once a week starting 1 week prior to the trip and ending 1 week after returning
D) Mefloquine once a week starting 1 week prior to the trip and ending 4 weeks after returning
E) Atovaquone-proguanil one day, during the trip and one week after returning.

218) Infection with each of the following can mimic Epstein-Barr (EBV) infectious mononucleosis EXCEPT:

A) Cytomegalovirus
B) Adenovirus
C) Human herpes virus (HHV) – 6
D) Paramyxovirus
E) Rubella

219) The medical and housekeeping staff liked your presentations so much; they have asked you to give a noon conference on safety precautions and infection control in the office setting. Each of the following is true statements regarding the handling of sharps in an office practice EXCEPT:

A) Do not recap the needles using two hands
B) Discard sharps yourself, even if an assistant is close by with closer access to the container
C) Discard sharps immediately after use in a nearby designated container
D) Discard the sharps container as soon as it is full
E) Make the sharp contents accessible to the staff but inaccessible to patients

220) **Which of the following is the most common cutaneous manifestation of secondary syphilis?**

A) Condylomata lata
B) Non-pruritic palmar maculopapules
C) Mocha latte
D) Palmar vesiculopustules
E) Emerson, Lake, and Palmar
F) Pruritic maculopapular rash

221) **Sensorineural hearing loss resulting from direct invasion of the inner ear is the most common manifestation of which of the following viral infections?**

A) Congenital CMV
B) Congenital HSV
C) Influenza
D) Rubeola
E) Coxsackie

222) **Which of the following complications of disseminated gonococcal infection would be likely in an adolescent girl?**

A) Meningitis
B) Hepatitis
C) Osteomyelitis
D) Perihepatitis
E) Endocarditis

223) **Waiting in your previously neat reception area are 50 to 100 students who recently helped clean up a park in Indiana. They also recently developed influenza-like syndrome including a low-grade fever, muscular aches, crackles on chest auscultation, and decreased appetite. The symptoms are probably a result of:**

A) Influenza
B) Coccidioidomycosis
C) Aspergillosis
D) Histoplasmosis
E) Hardus workus shockus

224) **A one month old is anemic, irritable, and noted to have skin lesions on the hands and feet. On physical examination, you also note hepatosplenomegaly and decreased movement of the extremities. Which of the following is the *most likely* diagnosis?**

A) Gonorrhea
B) Syphilis
C) Group B streptococcal infection
D) Cytomegalovirus infection
E) Toxoplasmosis

225) **You are evaluating an 8 year old boy who presents with fever, cough and malaise for 5 days. Chest x-ray shows bilateral diffuse infiltrates.**

The best treatment for this patient would be?

A) Supportive care including antipyretics
B) Supportive care including antipyretics and dextromethorphan
C) Azithromycin
D) Amoxicillin
E) Amoxicillin/clavulanic acid

226) Which of the following is true regarding the attending of day care by HIV positive students?

A) Full disclosure of the condition to the daycare center is mandatory by law
B) HIV positive students with eczema cannot attend
C) HIV positive students with occasional epistaxis cannot attend
D) HIV positive students with uncovered exudative skin lesions cannot attend
E) Non toilet trained HIV positive children must be kept separate from other children

227) Which of the following antibiotics would be the *best* choice in a 7 year old being treated with high dose amoxicillin for otitis media who is still symptomatic after 3 days of treatment and has a bulging erythematous tympanic membrane which does not move with insufflation?

A) Azithromycin
B) Higher dose amoxicillin
C) Amoxicillin clavulanic acid
D) Ciprofloxacin
E) Tetracycline

228) Each of the following antibiotics would be appropriate initial treatment in a patient suspected of having a skin infections caused by community acquired methicillin resistant Staph aureus *except:*

A) Amoxicillin/ clavulanic acid
B) Clindamycin
C) Trimethoprim/sulfamethoxazole
D) Linezolid
E) Vancomycin

229) Each of the following could be *a part of* prophylaxis for a male resident who examined the throat of a patient with a confirmed diagnosis of meningococcal sepsis (Serogroup A) *except?*

A) Rifampin 600 mg BID for 2 days
B) Rifampin 1200 mg q day for 4 days
C) Ceftriaxone 250 mg IM once
D) Ciprofloxacin 500 mg PO x 1
E) Meningococcal vaccine

230) Which of the following is true regarding Listeria monocytogenes infection?

A) Mothers of affected infants are always asymptomatic prior to delivery
B) Listerosis typically presents with monocytosis
C) The most common mode of transmission is via contaminated food
D) Listerosis typically presents with monocytopenia
E) Listeriosis typically presents with leukopenia

231) In addition to gentamicin, which of the following would be most appropriate to be used in a patient with Listeria monocytogenes meningitis who is allergic to penicillin?

A) Cefotaxime
B) Ceftriaxone
C) Trimethoprim-sulfamethoxazole
D) Chloramphenicol
E) Ampicillin

232) Which one of the following is most helpful in predicting poor neurodevelopmental outcome in an infant with congenital CMV disease?

A) Maternal IgM to CMV titers
B) Positive amnionic viral cultures
C) Positive polymerase chain reaction
D) Documented hearing deficit following maternal recurrent disease
E) Placental enlargement documented on ultrasound

233) You are caring for a child with cat scratch disease. The child is otherwise healthy with normal growth and development, immunizations up to date and no past history of recurrent infections. Which of the following is the most appropriate management?

A) Lymph node biopsy
B) Amoxicillin / clavulanic acid
C) Prednisone
D) Cephalexin
E) Supportive care and observation

234) Each of the following are true regarding the incubation period following a bite by a rabies infected animal *except:*

A) Incubation periods are longer in children
B) Incubation period are shorter in those on chronic steroids
C) Incubation periods are shorter with bites closer to the CNS
D) The mean incubation period is 30-90 days
E) The number of bites shortens the incubation period

235) **You are presented with a patient whose HBsAg, Total and IgM HBcAb all are positive. The HBsAb is negative. What is the correct interpretation of these results?**

A) Beam me up Scotty I have one for Mr. Spock
B) Immune after hepatitis B vaccination
C) Chronic hepatitis B infection
D) Acute hepatitis B infection
E) Immune after recovery from hepatitis B infection

236) **Which of the following is associated with a high hepatitis B viral replication rate?**

A) HBeAb
B) HBeAg
C) HBsAb with positive HBcAb
D) HBsAb with negative HBcAb
E) Helpmyeyesaresoglazedovermothshavebeenlandingonmyeyeswithoutmynoticing

237) **Which of the following is associated with immunity following recovery form hepatitis B infection?**

A) HBeAb
B) HBeAg
C) HBsAb with positive HBcAb
D) HBsAb with negative HBcAg
E) Howtheheckshouldlknow?

Metabolic

238) Each of the following metabolic disorders has an increased risk for cerebral vascular occlusion *EXCEPT* for:

A) Homocystinuria
B) Sulfite oxidase deficiency
C) Fabry's disease
D) Ornithine transcarbamylase deficiency
E) Tyrosinosis

239) All of the following are autosomal recessive disorders *EXCEPT* for:

A) Hunters syndrome
B) Hurlers syndrome
C) Tay Sachs disease
D) Wilson's disease
E) Kartagener's syndrome

240) In the following set of questions, decide if each numbered choice applies to (A) only, (B) only, both (C), or neither (D):

1) Course facies
2) Corneal clouding
3) Autosomal recessive
4) X-linked recessive
5) Skeletal involvement/ normal intelligence

(A) Hunters syndrome
(B) Hurlers syndrome
(C) Both
(D) Neither

241) A 6-month-old infant presents with developmental delay. The prenatal and delivery histories are both unremarkable. Initial development was normal.

However, the patient still has poor head control and the mother says he feels like "a jelly fish" without the container. The mother reports that the urine has taken on an odd odor and the initial hair was dark and is now much lighter. In addition to hypotonia, the physical exam is remarkable for weight in the 5%ile for age. Of the following, the most likely diagnosis in this clinical situation is:

A) Tyrosinase negative albinism
B) Galactosemia
C) Hereditary fructose intolerance
D) Tay Sachs disease
E) Phenylketonuria

242) Elevated serum ammonia levels would be seen with each of the following EXCEPT:

A) Reye's syndrome
B) Leigh disease
C) Liver failure
D) Methylmalonic academia
E) Ornithine transcarbamoylase deficiency

243) A 3-year-old boy with mental retardation is noted to have choreoathetoid movements, hyperreflexia, spasticity of the left leg, and positive Babinski's sign. There are signs of self-mutilation of the fingers and buccal mucosa. Which of the following is the *most likely* associated metabolic abnormality?

A) Increased BUN/Creatinine
B) Intracranial calcification
C) Increased urine organic acid concentration
D) Hypoglycemia
E) Increased serum uric acid concentration

244) You are evaluating a 4 month old baby because of generalized seizures. The infant has not gained weight or grown sufficiently. On physical examination you note hepatomegaly and a large abdomen in general. You note that the infant looks thin. Lab results are significant for hypoglycemia and elevated uric acid and lipid levels.

The most likely diagnosis is:

A) Van Gierke Disease
B) Pompe disease
C) Lesch- Nyhan syndrome
D) Congenital CMV infection
E) Congenital Toxoplasmosis

245) Which of the following is true regarding infants identified in newborn screening with elevated blood phenylalanine (PA) levels?

A) All of them have PKU on further testing
B) Most of them will have PKU
C) Most of them won't have PKU
D) Some will have biopterin deficiency
E) C and D

246) A 5 month old recently started on cereal presents with constipation and eyelids which remain open and have to be closed manually. There is evidence of decreased tone on physical exam. The anterior fontanelle is opened and normal size. Otherwise growth and development have been normal with no significant findings on newborn screening.

The most likely diagnosis is:

A) Myasthenia gravis
B) Maternal myasthenia gravis
C) Mitochondrial disorder
D) Botulism poisoning
E) Glycogen storage disease

247) You are evaluating a child who initially presented with tremors and anxiety. She now presents with hemolytic anemia, is icteric and with elevated PTT. Hepatomegaly is noted on physical exam.

Measurement of which of the following is likely to reveal the correct diagnosis?

A) Factor VIII levels
B) Platelet count
C) Liver function test
D) Serum ceruloplasmin
E) Indirect and direct bilirubin

Musculoskeletal

248) All of the following are true of, or associated with, Duchenne's muscular dystrophy *EXCEPT* for:

A) Pseudohypertrophy of the calves
B) It is inherited as an X-linked recessive trait
C) Gowers sign
D) Mother is always the asymptomatic carrier
E) Proximal muscle weakness

249) A 16 year old girl is referred to your office from her private high school because of "severe scoliosis" noted on routine screening. A 19-degree angle of thoracis scoliosis is noted.

Your note to the school nurse, confirms that you will:

A) Suggest physical therapy and twice weekly Rolfing massage at spa beach resort
B) Confirm the findings with MRI and refer to neurology for follow-up
C) Repeat films in 6 months
D) Repeat films in 2 years
E) Prescribe bracing and followup every 2 months

250) An 8 year old has had a decreased level of energy with a low-grade fever over the past 14 days. On physical exam you note that she is able to walk but is unable to run up flight of stairs and prefers to just lie down on the couch "like her father" according to the mother's description. You also note that her eyelids and cheeks have a reddish color to them. This disorder would *BEST* be treated with:

A) Antitoxin
B) Supportive measures
C) Steroids
D) Immunophoresis
E) IV gamma globulins

251) An 11-year-old soccer player sustained a Salter-Harris I fracture of his left ankle during a game yesterday. He injured the same ankle during a basketball game 9 months earlier. Which of the following is the *most likely* explanation for this child's current injury?

A) Incomplete healing of the old injury
B) Second unrelated injury
C) Osteolytic fracture
D) Osteochondritis dissecans
E) Conversion disorder

252) Each of the following is common findings with temporomandibular joint (TMJ) dysfunction EXCEPT:

A) Tinnitus
B) Preauricular pain
C) Otalgia in the absence of physical findings consistent with otitis media
D) Swelling of the TMJ
E) Decreased motion of the jaw

253) Each of the following is a risk factor for the development of slipped capital femoral epiphysis (SCFE) EXCEPT:

A) Hypothyroidism
B) Elevated estrogen levels
C) Elevated testosterone levels
D) Male gender
E) African-American

254) The *most common* benign bone tumor in children is:

A) Osgood-Schlatter's disease
B) Osteogenic sarcoma
C) Osteoid osteoma
D) Ewing's sarcoma
E) Osteochondroma

255) In counseling the parents of a child with achondroplasia, which of the following statements would be most appropriate?

A) The disorder is inherited as an autosomal recessive trait
B) Normal mental development is likely
C) Ventricular shunting will most likely be necessary
D) Bladder and bowel control is rarely affected
E) Chromosome analysis is indicated

256) You are evaluating a 3 year old boy who wakes up several times a week complaining of bilateral pain in his shins. He has not had a recent viral illness. He is afebrile and experiences no pain during the day. He is afebrile and there is no joint swelling, discoloration, or limited range of motion. There is no point tenderness and he is afebrile.

The most likely diagnosis is

A) Osteoid osteoma
B) Legg Calve Perthes
C) Toxic synovitis
D) Slipped capital femoral epiphysis
E) Growing pains

257) **Which of the following is true regarding Legg Calve Perthes disease?**

A) X-rays are more helpful and sensitive in detecting early disease
B) Onset after puberty carries a better prognosis
C) It frequently occurs in boys between ages 4-10
D) Boys tend to have a higher prevalence of bilateral disease
E) Bilateral disease is associated with more severe disease and a worse prognosis

258) **You are evaluating a limping 13 year old boy obese linebacker for his school team. He reports increasing left knee pain over 2 weeks which increased when he came down wrong on his ankle while playing basketball. While supine his leg is externally rotated and slightly flexed. You have a hard time internally rotating his hip secondary to pain. The most likely diagnosis is:**

A) Legg Calve Perthes
B) Osgood Schlatter
C) Slipped capital femoral epiphysis
D) Septic arthritis
E) Deep tissue hemangioma

259) **Idiopathic scoliosis in adolescents is:**

A) Inherited in an autosomal recessive pattern
B) X-linked dominant pattern
C) X-linked recessive pattern
D) Behavioral secondary to poor posture
E) Due to numerous factors

260) You are asked to diagnose a child suspected of having Duchenne muscular dystrophy. You will conduct the listed diagnostic studies in which order?

A) Muscle biopsy, genetic analysis , creatinine kinase levels
B) Muscle biopsy, creatinine kinase levels, genetic analysis
C) Genetic analysis, creatinine kinase levels , muscle biopsy
D) Creatinine kinase levels, genetic analysis, muscle biopsy
E) Creatinine kinase levels , muscle biopsy, genetic analysis

261) You are evaluating an infant with internally rotated feet. You correctly diagnose idiopathic talipes equinovarus (club foot) the most likely cause is:

A) Multifactorial
B) Fetal positioning
C) Normal finding
D) X-linked recessive inheritance
E) Autosomal recessive inheritance

262) Conservative management of congenital talipes equinovarus or club foot is:

A) A roundtrip ticket to club foot in the Caribbean
B) Physical therapy
C) Binding via tape
D) Casting and splinting
E) Muscle relaxants for 3 months

Neonatology

263) Which one of the following is a TRUE statement regarding *developmental dysplasia of the hip?* It is more common among:

A) African-American babies
B) The incidence is higher among males
C) There is no correlation with family history
D) It is associated with prematurity
E) It is associated with breech presentation

264) You are called to the delivery room to see a newborn with herniation of the abdominal contents. You note that a membrane covers the bowel contents. Which of the following is TRUE regarding omphaloceles?

A) They are a result of the failure of the umbilical ring to contract
B) They are rarely associated with other anomalies
C) They have been linked to a folate-deficient diet during pregnancy
D) It is associated with Beckwith-Wiedemann syndrome
E) Due to position, the membranous covering never ruptures during pregnancy

265) Each of the following newborn rashes requires nothing more than reassurance EXCEPT:

A) Erythema toxicum
B) Dry peeling skin
C) Miliaria crystalline
D) Midline lumbosacral skin tag
E) Yellow papules on the hard palate

266) Despite attempts to halt labor, a 28-week premature baby boy is born while you are on-call. You are paged to the DR. The FIRST thing you should do after delivery is:

A) Assess respiratory status and prepare for intubation
B) Provide positive pressure ventilation
C) Place infant on an open bed warmer as a source of radiant heat
D) Place oxygen saturation monitor on your finger tip with the alarm set for a saturation below 55% and a pulse greater than 375
E) Obtain oxygen saturation monitor reading and establish an airway

267) Much has been written about maternal-baby bonding. There have been an equal number of super bowl infomercials on male bonding and recent emphasis on father-infant bonding. The MOST important factor in predicting father child bonding is:

A) A father is more likely to engage in diaper changing activities[7] if they do not have to ask for "directions" to the diaper genie
B) Fathers are more likely to change their child's diapers regardless of gender if the diaper genie is shaped like one of the "Bud Bowl" players
C) How many times they watched the Dr. Phil show
D) Due to a smaller age gap, adolescent fathers are more likely to bond with their children regardless of their early interactions
E) The father's presence in the delivery room

268) A 5-week-old first-born male is presented to you with a history of projectile vomiting of increasing severity, now occurring after each meal. There is a history of pyloric stenosis in the family on the maternal side. The baby looks dehydrated and hungry. You palpate an olive on the abdominal exam, and the father, who happens to be a surgeon, notes that he felt the "pit" in the olive. Prior to making your brilliant diagnosis of pyloric stenosis, which will be confirmed on ultrasound, the lab values you will MOST LIKELY have to correct are:

A) Sodium 145, potassium 3.7, bicarb 24, chloride 100
B) Sodium 128, potassium 3.5, bicarb 35, chloride 87
C) Sodium 124, potassium 6.0, bicarb 20, chloride 90
D) Sodium 140, potassium 3.3, bicarb 25, chloride 108
E) Sodium 150, potassium 5.2, bicarb 10, chloride 124

---

[7] If not actual diaper changing.

269) Which of the following statements regarding pyloric stenosis is true?

A) It occurs more frequently in males regardless of birth order
B) It results in a metabolic hyperchloremic alkalosis
C) A skilled pediatrician can usually palpate the "olive" but only a skilled surgeon can feel the "pimento" in the olive
D) Post-op apnea is best prevented through pre-op rehydration and correction of metabolic alkalosis
E) The family history on the father's side is usually positive rarely on the maternal side

270) An infant is born to a mother who was treated for eclampsia. The Apgar scores were low, and the infant is noted to have poor tone with decreased deep tendon reflexes and lethargy. The infant's condition is *most likely* caused by:

A) Hypoglycemia
B) Hypocalcemia
C) Hypernatremia
D) Hypermanganesemia
E) Hypermagnesemia

271) At the routine 2-week visit, an infant is noted to have left-sided tilting of the head and a firm mass in the sternomastoid muscle on the left side. The *most appropriate* next step in the management would be:

A) Have the baby do the hokie pokie and turn his head around
B) Biopsy of the nodule
C) MRI of the head
D) EMG
E) Passive stretching exercise

272) A former ventilator-dependent premie with bronchopulmonary dysplasia (BPD) is admitted for a hernia repair. His routine medications include furosemide and potassium chloride supplements. You obtain an arterial blood gas and, with the infant on 40% oxygen, the results of the ABG are pH 7.49, PCO2 55 mm Hg, and PO2 90 mm HG. These findings are *best* explained by:

A) Nephrocalcinosis
B) Primary respiratory alkalosis
C) Furosemide-induced alkalosis
D) Appropriate for an infant with BPD
E) Most likely a result of lab error

273) A 4-month-old infant is referred to you by a family practitioner because of a bulging fontanelle and poor feeding.[8] The infant's parents insist on feeding "natural foods" and the "natural doctor" suggested they feed the infant large amounts of natural vitamin and mineral supplements, which they have done for over 3 weeks. An excess of which of the following would be *most likely* to cause the patient's symptoms?

A) Vitamin C
B) Manganese
C) Vitamin D
D) Zinc
E) Vitamin A

274) A newborn, born at 36 weeks gestation via an uneventful spontaneous vaginal delivery, develops progressive respiratory distress. Chest x-ray is remarkable for cardiomegaly as well as diffuse granular pattern and bilateral pleural effusions. At 3 hours of age, hypotension develops. The WBC is 3200. Which of the following is the *most likely* cause of this infant's respiratory problem?

A) Total anomalous pulmonary venous connection
B) Transient tachypnea of the newborn
C) Group B *Strep* pneumonia
D) RDS
E) Congenital pulmonary lymphangiectasia

---

[8] We're talking about the infant; the referring physician is fine.

275) You are evaluating a full term 3.6 kg boy in the delivery room born by repeat C/Section. The apgar scores were 7/9 and the respiratory rate is 80 with a heart rate of 160. The oxygen saturations dip to the low 90's on room air and the baby is given supplemental oxygen to maintain the saturations greater than 95% On the physical exam you note some mild subcostal retractions with good air movement. There are no cardiac murmurs noted. You order a CXR which reveals increased interstitial markings and fluid in some of the interlobar fissures.

The most likely diagnosis is:

A) Tetralogy of Fallot
B) Respiratory distress syndrome
C) Group B Strep pneumonia
D) Transient tachypnea of the newborn
E) Pulmonary hypertension

276) Approximately what percentage of newborns requires some form of resuscitation in the delivery room?

A) 1%
B) 10%
C) 25%
D) 50%
E) 65%

277) Within the first hour post delivery which of the following received top priority?

A) Vitamin K IM
B) Erythromycin ophthalmic ointment
C) Obtaining a weight
D) Measuring length
E) Allowing the infant to breast feed

278) Early discharge from the newborn nursery after a normal spontaneous vaginal delivery is considered prior to:

A) 12 hours
B) 24 hours
C) 48 hours
D) 72 hours
E) Depends on the HMO the parent's are enrolled in.

279) Infants must be seen within 48 hours if they are discharged prior to

A) 12 hours
B) 24 hours
C) 48 hours
D) 72 hours
E) Depends on the pediatrician

280) Breastfeeding jaundice commonly seen in the first 2-4 postnatal days is due to:

A) Decreased bilirubin conjugation
B) Decreased ligandin
C) IgA present in breast milk
D) Increased entero-hepatic circulation
E) Decreased entero-hepatic circulation

281) You are evaluating a 2 week old infant who is icteric. The baby is breastfeeding well and other than 3-4 clay colored stool per day he is doing well. On physical examination the baby is icteric with discoloration of the sclera and skin down to the pelvic area

The most likely explanation for the presentation is:

A) Breast feeding jaundice
B) Human milk associated jaundice
C) Cholestasis
D) Gilbert Syndrome
E) ABO incompatibility

282) Which of the following is true regarding conjugated hyperbilirubinemia?

A) It is just another name for direct hyperbilirubinemia
B) It is always associated with cholestasis
C) It is more common than unconjugated hyperbilirubinemia
D) It is defined as conjugated bilirubin greater than 2.0 or greater than 20% of the total bilirubin
E) Gilbert Syndrome results in unconjugated hyperbilirubinemia

283) You are called to the nursery to evaluate a 2.0 kg infant who was born at 36 weeks gestation 12 hours ago. The Apgar scores were 8/9. You confirm that the heart rate is 180/min. and the respiratory rate is 75/min. The MOST appropriate NEXT step would be to:

A) Obtain an EKG
B) Administer indomethacin
C) Obtain a serum blood glucose
D) Obtain serum lytes
E) Obtain a urine tox screen

284) You are evaluating a full-term infant that presents with noisy breathing and copious secretions requiring repeated suctioning from the oropharynx. The initial glucose water feeding results in a severe choking episode. The MOST appropriate next step would be to:

A) Ask the most experienced nurse to feed the infant and report results
B) Request a barium swallow examination
C) Obtain a CT of the head immediately
D) Insert a catheter into both nares to assure patency
E) Obtain an x-ray study of the chest after inserting a soft radiopaque feeding tube

285) Among the effects of terbutaline on a newborn includes each of the following EXCEPT:

A) Fetal hypoinsulinemia
B) Fetal hyperinsulinemia
C) Neonatal hyperglycemia
D) Fetal tachycardia
E) Hypotrophic cardiomyopathy

286) In addition to premature closure of the ductus arteriosus in the fetus exposed to indomethacin additional adverse effects include each of the following EXCEPT

    A) Irreversible renal failure
    B) Oligohydramnios
    C) Increased risk for periventricular leukomalacia
    D) Increased risk for necrotizing enterocolitis
    E) Reversible renal failure

287) Each of the following is true and/or associated with gastroesophageal reflux in infants *except:*

    A) Chronic wheezing
    B) Failure to thrive
    C) Head elevation in the supine position is always helpful
    D) Regurgitation often occurs 30 minutes after feeding
    E) Irritability during or after feedings

288) Each of the following is true of, or associated with rumination in infants *except:*

    A) Repeated and painless regurgitation
    B) Symptoms do not occur during sleep
    C) It does not respond to standard treatment for gastroesophageal reflux
    D) Symptoms must be present for 8 weeks or longer
    E) It is associated with retching

Neurology

289) Each of the following are associated with neurofibromatosis type 1 *EXCEPT* for:

A) Acoustic neuromas
B) Lisch nodules
C) Neurofibromas
D) Optic gliomas
E) Learning disabilities

290) Each of the following are true with regards to febrile seizures *EXCEPT*:

A) Neuroimaging is rarely indicated
B) The risk for developing epilepsy in a child who has experienced a febrile seizure is twice that of the general population
C) The risk of developing epilepsy is proportionate to the number of febrile seizures the child has experienced
D) Meningitis must be ruled out clinically in all cases
E) Serum electrolytes, glucose and calcium should not be ordered routinely

291) A 9year old is being seen in your office for a history of "staring spells" along with weird clicking sounds that some times lead to generalized seizures. After the episodes he is drowsy and out of it. The spells last a minute or two and 2 EEG's have been normal. A head CT, CBC and serum electrolytes are all unremarkable.

Your physical exam is unremarkable. There is no family history of seizures. This history is *most* consistent with a diagnosis of:

A) Absence seizures
B) Tourette's syndrome
C) Rolandic seizures
D) Partial seizures
E) Partial complex seizures

292) A 3 month old in your practice hasn't been eating well and is chronically lethargic. Head circumference is in the 96th percentile and weight is in the 6th percentile. Giving him the appearance of a Klingon on Star Trek the 2nd generation. Chest x- ray reveals significant cardiomegaly. A head CT with contrast reveals large ventricles with the 3rd ventricle compressed by a mass that is noted after contrast is given. This is confirmed by the radiologist who dictates this while taking a swig from her 5th triple mocha latte of the morning. You simultaneously shout out the *CORRECT* diagnosis:

A) Dandy Walker cyst
B) Epidural hematoma
C) VSD
D) Vein of Galen malformation
E) Subdural hematoma

293) **Match each number to its associated seizure on the right.**

1) 3 per second spike and wave EEG pattern   (A) Complex partial seizures
2) Hypsarrhythmia pattern on EEG   (B) Absence seizures
3) Lip smacking   (C) Infantile spasms
4) Occur at night   (D) Rolandic seizures

294) **Match each number to its corresponding dyskinesia on the right:**

1) Smooth movements of the extremities   (A) Chorea
2) Rhythmic movements of the head   (B) Dystonia
3) Twisting, assuming postures   (C) Hyperactivity
4) Brief muscle jerking movements   (D) Myoclonus
5) Brief movements of the face and shoulder   (E) Tics
6) Excessive ants-in-the-pants-like movements   (F) Tremor

295) A 15-year-old girl presents with a severe headache that began suddenly earlier today. The headache is severe and constant over the left side of her head. In addition, she is complaining about right-sided weakness, especially on the upper extremity. She has had no significant past history and takes no medication routinely. There is no family history of neurologic disease.

She is afebrile, and BP is 115/80 mm Hg. She is having difficulty with neck flexion, with positive Kernig and Brudzinski signs. She is lethargic and responds slowly to both verbal and visual stimuli. A right hemiparesis coupled with hyperreflexia is noted. Eye examination shows no papilledema, no evidence of a visual field deficit, and no sensory abnormalities. Head CT shows a hematoma in the posterolateral portion of the left frontal lobe. The MOST likely diagnosis is:

A) Cerebral aneurysm
B) Spinal meningitis
C) Subdural hematoma
D) Acute Encephalitis
E) Intracranial hemorrhage due to AV malformation

296a) A 9-year-old girl presents with progressive generalized weakness and increasing bilateral ptosis over the past 2-3 months. She presents in the emergency room because her symptoms have gotten worse over the past 2 days.

The parents note that the weakness gets worse over the course of the day. Fatigue sets in even with minimal physical activity. By evening her voice is weak and she has difficulty swallowing. Vision is normal except for occasional diplopia. The patient has had no fever, pain, rash, or joint swelling. She is receiving no medications.

Her birth history, prenatal history, and developmental history are all normal. Family history is negative for any neuromuscular disease.

On physical examination, you note mild bilateral ptosis, weakness of the left abducens nerve manifested by the inability to move the eye laterally, along with a diminished gag reflex. There is a nasal tone to her voice, suggesting laryngeal muscle weakness. She also has mild weakness of the extremities and notable muscle fatigue with repetitive tasks. CBC and differential are normal. The *most likely* diagnosis is:

A) Myasthenia gravis
B) Guillain-Barré syndrome
C) Multiple sclerosis
D) Botulism poisoning
E) Polio

296b) **This illness is due to:**

A) A virus
B) Antibodies
C) Myelin deterioration
D) Inhibition of neurotransmitter release
E) Toxin

296c) **The MOST appropriate management would be:**

A) Conservative management
B) Antibiotic therapy
C) Antiviral agents
D) Antitoxin
E) Cholinesterase inhibitors

297) A 6-month-old boy has been exhibiting abnormal movements and has been brought to you by the anxious parents. On physical examination, you note sudden flexion of the trunk as well as the neck and limbs. This is followed by gradual relaxation. EEG shows a hypsarrhythmic pattern. Of the following, the *most appropriate* treatment for this condition would be:

A) Phenytoin
B) Adrenocorticotropic hormone (ACTH)
C) Carbamazepine
D) Phenobarbital
E) Valproate

298) A 15-year-old boy is brought to the ED after his second major motor seizure. Physical examination shows a diminished sensorium and deviation of both eyes to the left. The BEST explanation for these findings is:

A) Postictal state
B) New York state of mind
C) Persistent seizure activity
D) Intranuclear ophthalmoplegia
E) Right-sided brain stem infarct

299) Early in an important high school game a 15-year-old hockey player in your practice is knocked unconscious after colliding with another player. He is "out" for approximately 2 minutes and afterward seems alert and oriented. He has had no previous injuries and is healthy. Results of a quick neurological examination are normal. He asks to return to the game. Assuming that this player continues to be asymptomatic and the head CT is normal, the most appropriate management in this situation is to allow him to return to play:

A) As soon as he is eligible for unrestricted free agency.
B) Immediately, without restrictions
C) Immediately, with the stipulation that he must come out every 5 minutes for reevaluation
D) After 1 day
E) After 1 week

300) A 10 year old girl presents with a history of a left sided headache along with paresthesias and weakness of the right arm and leg, preceding the headache she saw specks of light floating in her visual field. She has no difficulty speaking and the headache is still present during the exam. The mother notes that several members of her family suffer from severe migraine headaches.

The most likely diagnosis is

A) Confusional migraine
B) Basilar type migraine
C) Craniopharyngioma
D) Post viral labyrinthitis
E) Familial hemiplegic migraine

301) The parents of a 7 year old boy are concerned over a school report that describes several episodes where he turns his head followed by his eyes blinking. During the episodes he is fully aware of his surroundings and alert. The parents have also noticed similar episodes at home which occur on a daily basis.

In addition he has been noted to sniff during class which has continued despite being asked to stop on more than one occasion.

The most likely diagnosis would be:

A) Tic disorder
B) Tourette syndrome
C) Absence seizures
D) Attention deficit hyperactivity disorder
E) Allergic rhinitis

302) Which one of the following is true regarding teenagers with a history of epilepsy?

A) Bathing in a tub or swimming is prohibited
B) Before withdrawing from medications a normal baseline EEG must be obtained
C) Juvenile myoclonic epilepsy requires lifetime treatment
D) Driving is prohibited in any teenager treated for epilepsy
E) Driving is acceptable if seizure free for at least 24 months while on anticonvulsants

303) You are caring for a child experiencing a febrile seizure for the first time. Which one of the following would be considered to be risk factors for subsequently developing epilepsy?

A) Onset of febrile seizure before age 1
B) Low degree of fever at the onset of the seizure
C) Family history of febrile seizures
D) Family history of epilepsy
E) Male gender

Nutrition

304) Which of the following statements regarding breast-feeding is *TRUE?*

A) Breast-feeding through the first 6 months of life is adequate
B) The components of breast milk remain constant through the first year
C) Breast milk provides protection against infection primarily through IgG and passive immunity
D) Human milk contains activated T cells and alpha interferon
E) Human milk likely complements the infant's own immune system via immunomodulation.

305) During the first 6 months of life, which of the following can be obtained exclusively with breast milk under *ALL* conditions?

A) Phylloquinone
B) Fluoride
C) Vitamin D
D) Ascorbic Acid
E) Vitamin B12

306) Match the numbered descriptions on the left with the forms of Vitamin D on the right.

1) Ergocalciferol
2) Cholecalciferol
3) Hydroxylated in the liver
4) Activated calcitriol
5) Hydroxylated in the kidney

(A) 1,25 hydroxy vitamin D
(B) 25, hydroxy vitamin D
(C) Vitamin D_2
(D) Vitamin D_3

307) **Match the clinical manifestations on the left with the deficiency on the right.**

1) Scaly dermatitis, alopecia, thrombocytopenia
2) Dry skin, poor wound healing, perioral rash
3) Hemolytic anemia, peripheral edema, thrombocytopenia

(A) Zinc deficiency
(B) Vitamin E deficiency
(C) Essential fatty acid deficiency
(D) Ascorbic acid deficiency

308) **Regarding protocol in the *United States*, what would be the most appropriate nutrition to provide to a child born to a mother who is HIV-positive?**

A) Breast feeding
B) Commercially prepared formula
C) Filtered mother's breast milk
D) Mother's breast milk after freezing[9]
E) Irradiated breast milk
F) Pooled breast milk

309) **Which of the following is TRUE regarding medium chain triglycerides?**

A) They are not present in human milk
B) They are not present in cow's milk
C) They are never present in commercially available infant formula
D) They require micelle formation with bile salts for adequate absorption
E) They are obtained by chopping triglycerides using a "medium-sized chain-saw"

310) **Deficiency of biotin results in:**

A) Seborrhea
B) Keratomalacia
C) Glossitis
D) Oxaluria
E) Sensory neuropathy

---

[9] Freezing the milk, not the mother or her breast.

311) Oxaluria would *most likely* be the result of the EXCESS of which of the following?

A) Niacin
B) Ascorbic acid
C) Riboflavin
D) Cyanocobalamin
E) Retinol

312) An adolescent girl following a strict vegan diet is most likely to develop deficiency of which of the following water-soluble vitamins?

A) Folic acid
B) Niacin
C) Riboflavin
D) Cobalamin
E) Thiamine

313) You are evaluating a child of a 6 year old child recently adopted from China. The parents are very concerned because the child seems to bump into objects in the evening after he has completed his homework and is getting ready for bed.

The teachers state that he has no similar difficulty at school. He is below the 25th percentile for weight and height. On physical examination he is noted to have skin which is dry and scaly. In addition silver patches are noted on his conjunctiva. What is the most likely explanation for the child's clinical presentation?

A) Tocopherol deficiency
B) Attention deficit hyperactivity disorder
C) Retinol deficiency
D) Chronic use of methylphenidate
E) Psoriasis

314) You are asked to evaluate a 9 month old white male who has been breast fed exclusively. He has had recurrent episodes of bronchiolitis treated with albuterol. Recently he has had bouts of foul smelling diarrhea.

On physical exam the child appears to be fussy with decreased muscle tone. His conjunctiva are mildly injected. His labs findings include low serum calcium elevated alkaline phosphatase and anemia with a slight increase in indirect bilirubin.

Which of the following would be the most likely explanation for *all* of the clinical findings?

A) Vitamin D deficiency
B) Vitamin E deficiency
C) Vitamin A deficiency
D) Poor exposure to UV light
E) Cystic fibrosis

315) You are evaluating a one week old boy who is visiting from out of town. He has been exclusively breast-fed. You note mild bleeding from nares, the umbilical stump as well as the circumcision site. The infant has not been seen by his pediatrician or any other clinician other than the nurse midwife who delivered the baby at home.

The most appropriate treatment of this baby will be:

A) Vitamin K, 2 units
B) Fresh frozen plasma
C) Van Willebrand Factor
D) Factor 8
E) Factor 9

316) Which of the following is true regarding the caloric needs of full term vs. preterm infants?

A) Full term infants require 100- 120 Kcal / Kg / day
B) Preterm infants require 100- 120 Kcal/ Kg/ day
C) A and B
D) Full term infants require a minimum 150 Kcal/Kg/day
E) Preterm infants require 80-100 Kcal/Kg/ day

317) You are managing a severely malnourished 16 year old female admitted for management of anorexia nervosa. She must be medically cleared before receiving psychiatric treatment. During refeeding the electrolyte abnormality during the first week of treatment that you should be most concerned about would be:

A) Hyperphosphatemia
B) Hypophosphatemia
C) Hypocalcemia
D) Hypercalcemia
E) Hypernatremia

318) You are taking care of a one month old who has a documented gram negative sepsis. Additional findings include hepatomegaly, elevated indirect bilirubin and positive reducing substances in the stool.

The most likely explanation for this infant's clinical presentation would be:

A) Congenital toxoplasmosis infection
B) G6PD deficiency
C) Galactose-1-phosphate uridyltransferase deficiency
D) 21-hydroxylase deficiency
E) Congenital cytomegalovirus infection

Pharmacology

319) In the following set of questions, for each numbered word or phrase, choose the lettered heading that is MOST CLOSELY ASSOCIATED with it. Lettered headings may be selected once, more than once, or not at all.

1) Metabolic acidosis
2) Hypokalemic alkalosis
3) Contraction alkalosis
4) Potassium sparing

(A) Furosemide
(B) Acetazolamide
(C) Spironolactone
(D) Hydrochlorothiazide

320) **Trimethoprim/ Sulfamethoxazole would be the first line treatment for each of the following EXCEPT :**

A) Pneumocystis carinii pneumonia prophylaxis
B) urinary tract infection prophylaxis
C) urinary tract infection due to enterococcus
D) Listeria monocytogenes in penicillin allergic patients
E) exacerbation of chronic bronchitis

321) **Which of the following medications should be used with caution when taking sedatives?**

A) Echinacea
B) Ginseng
C) Valerian Root
D) St. John's Wort
E) Peppermint Patty

322) **Which of the following medications is postulated to act by inhibiting serotonin reuptake?**

A) Echinacea
B) Ginseng
C) St. Johns' Wort
D) Valerian Root
E) St. John's Band

323) **Match each number (chemotherapeutic agent) to its associated *toxicity* on the right.**

1) Cyclophosphamide
2) Bleomycin
3) Doxorubicin
4) Anthracycline
5) Vincristine
6) Asparaginase
7) Methotrexate

(A) Cardiac toxicity
(B) CNS problems
(C) Hemorrhagic cystitis
(D) Neurotoxicity
(E) Oral ulcerations
(F) Pancreatitis
(G) Pulmonary fibrosis

Preventive

324) **Regarding childhood drowning, each of the following are true EXCEPT:**

A) Drowning occurs more frequently in boys than girls
B) If swimming pools are excluded; those of lower socioeconomic status are at greater risk of drowning
C) Toddlers between the ages of 1 and 3 are at the greatest risk for drowning
D) Infant and toddler swimming lessons reduce the risk for drowning
E) A fence that surrounds and separates the pool from the house and yard significantly reduces the risk for drowning

325) **You have been asked to give a talk to a group of new parents on preventing injuries. You are asked: "what is the most common way in which children receive burn injuries?" You correctly answer:**

A) Matches
B) Flames
C) Electrical wires
D) Hot liquids
E) Radiators

326) **Which one of the following statements is TRUE?**

A) Dietary sugar is often a contributing factor to hyperactive behavior in children
B) When used in combination, acetaminophen and ibuprofen are more effective in reducing fever than when either is used alone
C) A 12-day course of steroids for acute asthma should be tapered
D) To accelerate healing and decrease irritation, corneal abrasions must be patched in addition to using topical antibiotic
E) Going out with wet hair can affect immunity and lead to increased risk of pneumonia

327) **A 7-week-old infant in your practice develops a documented case of pertussis. The BEST treatment for his 6-1/2-year-old brother, who has received 5 doses of DTaP, the most recent one 2 years ago, would consist of:**

A) A DTaP booster and a 14-day course of erythromycin
B) No additional immunizations, and but a 14-day course of erythromycin
C) No additional immunizations, but a 14-day course of erythromycin at the start of any clinical sign
D) No additional immunizations, but a 10-day course of erythromycin
E) A DTaP booster and a 5-day course of clarithromycin

328) **All of the following are possible reactions to the varicella vaccine EXCEPT for:**

A) Death
B) Anaphylaxis
C) Temporal lobe seizure
D) Encephalitis
E) ITP

329) **Varicella vaccine is contraindicated in each of the following situations EXCEPT:**

A) Children with a history of an anaphylactic reaction to gelatin or neomycin
B) Pregnant women
C) Children receiving high-dose corticosteroids for more than 2 weeks
D) HIV patients who are mildly symptomatic
E) Children with acute lymphocytic leukemia who are not in remission

330) Which of the following BEST describes a possible side effect of the varicella vaccine?

A) High fever
B) Necrotizing fascitis
C) Acute cerebellar ataxia
D) Seizures
E) *Streptococcus pyogenes* infection at the injection site

331) Which of the following is TRUE regarding cholesterol screening and promoting healthy cholesterol levels in children?

A) Egg whites should be substituted for fats
B) Total cholesterol or HDL levels require fasting
C) Calculation of LDL cholesterol levels does not require fasting
D) Cholesterol levels decrease before puberty and rapidly increase during the growth spurt.
E) Changing to low-fat dairy products is sufficient for children younger than 2 years of age.

332) An investigator compares the results of laboratory tests with the presence of a disease and tabulates the results as follows:

Test Results	With Disease	Without Disease
Positive	81	5
Negative	37	48

The investigator reports that 0.68 is the:

A) Sensitivity of the test
B) Specificity of the test
C) Prevalence of the test
D) Accuracy of the test
E) Positive predictive value for the test

333) An investigator compares the results of laboratory testing with the presence of a disease and tabulates the results as follows

Test Results	With Disease	Without Disease
Positive	81	5
Negative	37	48

The investigator reports that 0.90 is the:

A) Sensitivity of the test
B) Specificity of the test
C) Prevalence of the test
D) Accuracy of the test
E) Positive predictive value for the test

334) An investigator compares the results of laboratory testing with the presence of a disease and tabulates the results as follows:

Test Results	With Disease	Without Disease
Positive	81	5
Negative	37	48

The investigator reports that 0.94 is the:

A) Sensitivity of the test
B) Specificity of the test
C) Prevalence of the test
D) Accuracy of the test
E) Positive predictive value for the test

Psychosocial

335) His mother, a VP for a venture capital group, brings Johnny Edhopperman to your ER. You are in the middle of your 89-hour shift in central Connecticut. Mom is exasperated because her child has been vomiting for 6 months and none of the doctors who work in "the City" have done anything.

The mother calmly tells you to "look at my son; he is clearly hypovolemic, dry and his cap refill is 3 seconds or more. Please help him." After obtaining electrolytes and giving him several normal saline boluses, which additional lab should you order to clinch the diagnosis for this mother?

A) Maternal porcelain levels
B) Serum emetine levels
C) No labs. Ask the mother to prepare a press release since the workup was all wrong and the public needs to know
D) CBC, Diff, Blood Culture and ESR

336) In the following set of questions, decide if each numbered choice applies to (A) only, (B) only, both (C), or neither (D):

1) First third of the night
2) Enuresis
3) Mobile during episode
4) Recall of episode
5) Positive family history
6) Tucker Carlson as president

(A) Night terrors
(B) Nightmares
(C) Both
(D) Neither

337) An 8-year-old boy with ADHD is brought for routine evaluation. His parents want to know about appropriate dietary therapy. Which of the following is the BEST advice based upon the latest research?

A) Restrict all foods that contain sugar
B) Eliminate all foods that contain artificial coloring and artificial preservatives
C) Eliminate all processed foods
D) Eat whatever he wants
E) Eat a well balanced diet; ADHD has no relation to diet

338) A 2-1/2-year-old boy is brought to your office for a routine visit. The parents notice that he will often repeat the first word in a sentence, especially when he is rushed or tired. Although it doesn't occur all the time, it does occur when the child is asked a question. You should:

A) Order a neurological workup
B) Obtain a formal hearing evaluation
C) Refer the child for speech therapy
D) Rule out ankyloglossia
E) Reassure the mother

339) Which of the following would be reasonable expectations of a child with an IQ of 70?

A) Achieve academic skill levels of a 7th grader
B) Some vocational skills while living at a supervised group home
C) Marry and become a successful parent
D) Communication skills development in the preschool years
E) Become a political pundit on their own show Sunday mornings on major network

340) The most common presentation of mental retardation is:

A) Delayed motor development
B) Poor social skills
C) Reading disability
D) Language delay
E) Seizures

341) Each one of the following is a true statement regarding primitive reflexes EXCEPT:

A) They are normal in infants but abnormal in others
B) They are brainstem-mediated
C) They disappear during the first year as voluntary motor activity emerges
D) Corneal reflex is an example
E) Step reflex is an example
F) They are never normal in adult males

342) An 18-month-old former 24-week premie is being seen for a routine well-baby visit. The child was ventilator-dependent for one month, with head ultrasounds, hearing screens, and eye exams all normal. The mother is concerned because of the lack of speech development. You note that the baby seems to respond to a one-step verbal command and can wave goodbye. She uses one-syllable words to express herself in addition to *dada* and *mama*. You should:

A) Reassure the mother
B) Head CT to rule out any head bleed that was missed initially
C) Repeat the hearing test
D) Refer to a speech pathologist
E) She is past the time when prematurity would account for the delay

343) You need to evaluate an 18 month year old boy because his parents are concerned about his tendency to bang his head and suck his thumb especially before going to bed. His growth and development are otherwise normal.

The most likely diagnosis is

A) Tourette Syndrome
B) Rett syndrome
C) Pervasive developmental disorder
D) Autism
E) Normal developmental variant

344) The parents of a 9-year-old boy report being awakened by a panicky scream coming from their child's room roughly 2 hours after he fell asleep. They were unable to console him or wake him up. When they arrived in his room he was tachycardic and tachypneic and eventually calmed down. He was unable to recall the event in the morning. You should advise them that this is MOST likely due to:

A) Watching American idol earlier
B) Nightmare
C) Night terror
D) Rolandic epilepsy
E) Anxiety disorder

345) An 8-year-old child is brought to your practice because of his inability to "stay on task" at school and his banter with the kids in the back of the room where he sits. When asked what the problem is, he tells you *"I'm sorry I wasn't listening".* The parents state there is nothing wrong and all he needs is a tutor.

They note that his dad, a trader on the NY stock exchange making millions had the same difficulty when he was a child. Your BEST approach to the problem is:

A) Ask dad if he would be willing to train you to work on the floor of the exchange as his protégé.
B) Explain that the beneficial effects of stimulant meds are almost immediate, and write a script for 5 mg methylphenidate q AM with followup in one week.
C) Explain that the beneficial effects of stimulant meds are evident, and write a script for 5 mg methylphenidate q AM for 3 days followed by 10 mg dexmethylphenidate XR q day if it is working, with followup in a week.
D) Explain the possibility of a diagnosis of ADD and that the diagnosis does not carry a poor prognosis. Offer literature on the subject and suggest a followup visit in a week.
E) Write a script for methylphenidate 5 mg, schedule an appointment for psychological testing to rule out a learning disorder, and suggest that he be seated in the front of the room where there is less distraction.

346) The mother of a 15-month-old infant states that he eats table food but "drinks nothing but a pint of milk" each day. Weight and length are at the 25%. Weight and height percentiles were the same at 9 months of age. The most important thing to do at this time is to:

A) Order a UA and determine the serum BUN
B) Suggest increasing the caloric density of the infant's diet
C) Reassure the mother that growth and eating habits are within normal limits for this period of life
D) Plan an elective hospitalization to evaluate his failure to thrive
E) Prescribe an appetite stimulant

347) A 7-year-old boy is evaluated because of a recent deterioration in school performance. Medical history is unremarkable except for hydronephrosis with associated infection for which he received a 1-month course of aminoglycoside therapy 6 months ago. Which of the following is the most likely cause of this boy's academic problems?

A) Focal brain abscess
B) Progressive uremia
C) ADHD
D) Temporal lobe seizures
E) Hearing loss

348) An infant sits comfortably on your examining table, and his back is straight. He takes a stick from your hand, using a pincer grasp, and transfers it to his other hand. He smiles, showing two teeth. His mother reports that he crawls. He does not pull himself to a standing position, but he supports his weight and takes tentative and clumsy steps with both hands held. The developmental age of this infant is closest to:

A) 6 months
B) 9 months
C) 12 months
D) 15 months
E) Indeterminate without additional data

349) An 11-year-old boy is being evaluated because his teachers do not think that his school performance matches his ability. His birth history is normal.

His teachers report that he leaves his seat at inappropriate times and talks excessively during class. The parents assume that their son will eventually outgrow this "adjustment period".

His school performance has declined steadily for the past 2 years, which his teachers attribute to difficulty completing assignments and homework. General physical findings are normal. The boy is well behaved but fidgety. Neurologic evaluation is normal. He has well-coordinated gross and fine motor movements.

When you evaluate him he focuses well and pays attention. Which of the following is the most likely diagnosis?

A) Oppositional defiant disorder
B) Mental retardation
C) Gilles de la Tourette syndrome
D) Normal developmental period
E) Attention deficit hyperactivity disorder

350) You are evaluating a 2 year old for a well visit. The mother is a single mother, there during her lunch hour and is breast feeding her 6 month old. Her 4 year old other child is in the waiting room playing. The mother had to go out several times to attend to the 4 year old who was fighting with another child in the waiting room play area.

She is awaiting the arrival of their part time nanny who takes over at lunch. The mother works out of their home office and watches the patient and their other two children while working out of her home office as a paralegal.

What would you suggest for this mother?

A) Offer her additional work as a paralegal
B) Refer her for social work consultation
C) Suggest that she work at night
D) Suggest that she incorporate the 4 year old into her work routine
E) That she is doing a fine job juggling her responsibilities.

351) Each of the following is true regarding families with a child with a chronic illness *except:*

A) Children with special needs are at increased risk for physical abuse and neglect at home
B) Children with special needs are at increased risk for physical abuse and neglect in educational and child care settings
C) The divorce rate is the same as in families without a child with a special need
D) Family members are at increased risk for depression

352) Which of the following is the most likely cause of a 6 week old infant who cries 3 hours a day and is growth and development are normal. The crying occurs suddenly, is persistent, and can last for more than one hour

A) The need to change formula
B) The need for the breastfeeding mother to monitor her diet closely
C) Infantile colic
D) Tntussusception
E) Reflux esophagitis

353) Which of the following is true regarding TV watching in children?

A) More than 50% of parents enforce TV viewing limits
B) Less than 50% of homes of children 8 years and older have the TV on during meals
C) 25% of children 8 years and older have video games in their room
D) 25% of children 8 years and older have TV's in their rooms
E) The AAP recommends that children younger than 2 years of age should watch no TV

354) Which of the following are most effective in pediatric patients requiring pharmacological treatment of separation anxiety disorder?

A) Desipramine
B) Atomoxetine
C) Fluoxetine
D) Clonazepam
E) Risperidone

Pulmonary

355) Bronchiectasis is best diagnosed by:

A) Serial chest X rays
B) Arteriography
C) Pulmonary function testing
D) CT scan
E) Radionucleotide study

356) A 6-month-old infant former 27 week preemie is failing to thrive (FTT). Caloric intake is adequate. Medications include multivitamins and albuterol. The infant was weaned from oxygen therapy 2 months ago. Vital signs are normal and the physical examination is normal except for FTT. CXR findings are consistent with bronchopulmonary dysplasia. Which of the following is the next appropriate step?

A) Measure oxygen SATs while the infant is sleeping
B) Restart oxygen therapy
C) Start Pulmicort® twice a day via nebulizer
D) Sweat chloride
E) Reassure the mother that this is expected with bronchopulmonary dysplasia

357a) A 5-year-old boy presents with 5 months of intermittent fever, fatigue, and weight loss accompanied by coughing. He has just completed a course of amoxicillin with minimal improvement. His appetite and PO intake have been poor. He has a past medical history significant for several upper respiratory infections as well as several bouts of otitis media. His immunizations are all up to date.

According to his mother he has had fever for 5 weeks, the mother notes that she too has had a nagging cough for several months. The boy has had no other associated symptoms such as vomiting, diarrhea, urinary problems, or rash.

On physical examination, his temperature is 38.5 C and his vital signs are stable. HEENT exam is normal except for several palpable 1-cm anterior cervical lymph nodes. Examination of the lungs reveals wheezes and crackles on the right. Physical examination is otherwise normal.

Labs: H/H 32/14, WBC 5, 60 P, 30 L, 10 M, MCV 80, platelets 450, ESR 50, CXR-R perihilar infiltrate, with hilar adenopathy. The *most likely* diagnosis is:

A) *Staph aureus* pneumonia
B) Pneumococcal pneumonia
C) RSV bronchiolitis
D) Reactive airway disease
E) Pneumonia secondary to *Mycobacterium tuberculosis*

357b) The most appropriate next step in confirming the diagnosis would be:

A) CBC and blood culture
B) Switching antibiotics
C) PPD placement
D) RSV screening
E) Open lung biopsy

126

358) A 6-week-old is brought to the ER for evaluation of "noisy breathing" and "choking". The mother notes that this has been going on since birth and their pediatrician has done nothing. She wants you to do something right now!

Growth and development are normal. The infant breast-feeds well. On physical examination, intermittent mild intercostal and subcostal retractions and mild inspiratory stridor are present. There are no wheezing, rales or rhonchi. Which of the following is the *most appropriate* next course of action?

A) pH probe study
B) Reassurance
C) Inspiratory and expiratory x-ray studies of the chest
D) Call the pediatrician at home and ask how he can sleep knowing this child is suffering like this.
E) Pulse oximetry

359) You are evaluating a 9-month-old whose mother claims is "always sick". Which of the following would lead you to believe that this is something more than a routine upper respiratory tract infection that would suggest a possible immunodeficiency?

A) Ten upper respiratory tract infections during the past 6 months
B) Serial episodes of bilateral otitis media
C) Recurrent "pneumonia" with wheezing
D) Two hospitalizations for febrile pneumonia
E) Severe post-tussive emesis

360) You are called to evaluate an infant in the nursery who becomes cyanotic at rest. The cyanosis clears up with vigorous crying. You suspect a diagnosis of choanal atresia. All of the following are true EXCEPT:

A) Diagnosis is made by the failure to pass an NG tube by more than 2 trained personnel.
B) It is associated with cardiac malformations
C) It is associated with ear anomalies.
D) Obstruction of both nares can be life threatening in an infant younger than 5 months
E) Initial treatment is with an oropharyngeal airway.

361) A diagnosis of exercise-induced asthma is supported by a decrease in the forced expiratory volume (FEV$_1$) by at least:

A) 2%
B) 5%
C) 15%
D) 35%
E) 50%
F) 75%

362) A 12-year-old girl, diagnosed with asthma at age 2, is here for a routine evaluation. Her symptoms are worse at night, although she sometimes wheezes and coughs during the day. She does have periods where she is asymptomatic. Appropriate management would consist of each of the following EXCEPT:

A) Steroids twice a day delivered via a nebulizer
B) Albuterol 3 times a day via a nebulizer
C) Albuterol 4 times a day as needed for cough and wheeze
D) Instructions on use of peak flow meter
E) Intranasal steroids

363) Each of the following is true regarding inhaled corticosteroids used in the treatment of asthma EXCEPT:

A) They induce the production of beta 2 receptors, enhancing action of beta 2 agonists such as albuterol
B) They reduce the number of mast cells in cells lining the airway.
C) They decrease the synthesis of leukocyte protease inhibitor.
D) As many as 50% of patients who are well controlled with inhaled corticosteroids can still experience exercise-induced asthma.
E) With a conventional metered dose inhaler, 80%-90% of the inhaled dose is deposited in the oropharynx.

364) The mother of a 9-year-old child reports that he has had at least twelve episodes of "pneumonia" in the fall and winter seasons over the past 4 years. Between episodes, she says that he seems to be healthy, although he has frequent episodes of coughing. His height and weight are at the 30% for age. Scattered, low-pitched wheezes are heard in all lung fields on forced expiration. Findings on x-ray study of the chest are normal except for partial right middle lobe atelectasis. Which of the following is the most likely diagnosis?

A) Reactive airway disease
B) Cystic fibrosis
C) Foreign body aspiration
D) Tension pneumothorax
E) Congenital absence of the secretory component of IgA

365) A patient with acute asthma is most likely to have decreased:

A) Peak expiratory flow rate
B) Residual volume
C) Functional residual capacity
D) Total lung capacity
E) Tidal volume

366) Which of the following statements is true regarding the treatment of acute asthma exacerbations in children?

A) Levalbuterol has not been proven to be superior to racemic albuterol as a first line bronchodilator
B) Bacterial infections are implicated much more commonly as triggers than viral infections
C) It is never appropriate to have a patient maintain a supply of systemic steroids
D) Chest physical therapy should be a part of routine care in asthma exacerbations
E) Inhaled mucolytics should be a part of routine care in asthma exacerbations

367) Which of the following describes a patient with *mild intermittent* asthma?

A) General symptoms and night symptoms less than 2 times a week
B) General symptoms and night symptoms less than 2 times a month
C) General symptoms less than 2 times a week with night symptoms less than 2 times a month
D) General symptoms less than 2 times a month and night symptoms less than 2 times a week
E) General symptoms and night symptoms less than 2 times a month

368) Each of the following are appropriate treatment options in children with *moderate persistent asthma* except?

A) Medium dose inhaled steroid plus a long acting bronchodilator
B) Medium dose inhaled steroid alone
C) Medium dose inhaled steroid and a leukotriene modifier
D) Medium dose inhaled steroid and theophylline
E) Inhaled Cromolyn Sodium alone

369) Each of the following statements is true regarding the mechanism of action of pharmacological agents used to treat asthma *except:*

A) Inhaled cromolyn prevents both the early and late airway response to *allergy triggered* asthma
B) Inhaled steroids help inhibit the late but not the late bronchospastic response
C) Severe early bronchospasm responds promptly to short acting bronchodilators
D) Mast cell activation is responsible for the late bronchospastic response to allergen exposure.
E) Inflammation is the underlying abnormality present in patients who have even mild asthma.

370) You are evaluating a 7 year old with general malaise, low grade fever, headache and dry cough. Chest x-ray reveals bilateral patchy infiltrates. The most likely diagnosis would be:

A) Acute smoke inhalation
B) Bordetella pertussis
C) Bodega pertussis
D) Mycoplasma pneumonia
E) RSV pneumonia

Renal

371) All of the following causes of glomerulonephritis are accompanied by low serum complement levels *EXCEPT* for:

A) Post-strep glomerulonephritis
B) Membranoproliferative glomerulonephritis
C) Systemic lupus nephritis
D) Rapidly progressive glomerulonephritis

372) Each of the following are associated with medullary cystic kidney disease in children EXCEPT:

A) Acute onset
B) Polyuria
C) Polydipsia
D) Anemia
E) Growth failure

373) A 16-year-old boy is seeing you for a pre-sports physical. His previous physical exams and laboratory findings have been within normal limits. His father and uncle both have hypertension. His blood pressure, taken on 3 separate occasions over one hour, was between 140/90 mm Hg and 145/95 mm Hg. BP in the left leg was 150/100. Urinalysis, CBC, and renal studies were all within normal limits. Of the following, the MOST likely diagnosis is:

A) Renal vascular disease
B) Post strep glomerulonephritis
C) Pheochromocytoma
D) Essential hypertension
E) Hyperthyroidism

374) Each of the following are associated with prune belly syndrome EXCEPT:

A) Cryptorchidism (in males)
B) Ovarian dysplasia (in females)
C) Decreased muscle fiber in the urinary tract
D) Pulmonary hypoplasia
E) Renal dysplasia

375) A 6-year-old child is transferred to your practice because the parents are not happy with the care he has received elsewhere. The child is in the 4th percentile for both height and weight.[10] Lab results show Sodium of 136, Potassium of 3.2, Chloride of 114, and a serum Bicarb of 10. The Urine pH is 6.7. You win the parents over by noting that the MOST likely diagnosis based on these findings is:

A) Polycystic kidney disease
B) Congenital short stature
C) Metabolic organic acidosis
D) Distal tubular acidosis
E) Proximal tubular acidosis

376) A 4-year-old presents with periorbital and pretibial edema. Blood pressure is noted to be 130/85. Lab results include a BUN of 30, creatinine of 1.2, and albumin of 1.6. The MOST likely diagnosis based on these findings would be:

A) Focal segmental glomerulonephritis
B) Minimal change nephrotic syndrome
C) Lupus nephritis
D) Liver failure
E) Henoch-Schönlein purpura

---

[10] And the parents are in the 95%ile for anger.

377) An 8-year-old girl presents with a history of dysuria for 2 to 3 days. She is afebrile. The urinalysis reveals a urine pH of 8.0 with 4-5 RBC and 10-15 WBC. The MOST likely organism causing the UTI would be:

A) E. Coli
B) Proteus
C) Tuberculosis
D) Viral
E) Klebsiella

378) In addition to an infectious etiology, hemolytic uremic syndrome can also be caused by each of the following EXCEPT:

A) Inborn error of cobalamin metabolism
B) Autosomal recessive inheritance
C) Pregnancy
D) X-linked recessive inheritance pattern
E) Oral contraceptive use

379) While hematuria is often a benign incidental finding in children, it can sometimes indicate a glomerular lesion. Which of the following is TRUE regarding hematuria and glomerular disease?

A) Urine is tea-colored and actually contains tea leaves
B) The absence of dysmorphic RBCs all but rules out glomerular disease
C) The presence of casts containing RBCs is the most ominous sign
D) The presence of serrated RBCs in urinary sediment is the most ominous sign.
E) A 24-hour calcium/creatinine is required to rule out hypercalciuria as the cause of hematuria.

380) Each of the following renal stones can be seen in plain x-ray *except*

A) Calcium
B) Oxalate
C) Struvite
D) Uric acid
E) Cystine

381) Which of the following imaging studies offers the highest sensitivity and specificity in identifying renal stones of various composition and size?

A) Renal Ultrasound
B) IVP
C) Helical nonenhanced CT
D) Helical enhanced CT
E) Plain x-ray

382) Each of the following is true regarding cystine renal stones *except:*

A) Recurrent nephrolithiasis is the only clinical manifestation of cystinuria
B) Cystinuria can be associated with calcium oxalate stones
C) Cystinosis is associated with nephrolithiasis
D) Urine alkalization is part of the treatment
E) Increased fluid intake is part of the treatment

383) Routine ultrasound during pregnancy reveals severe oligohydramnios and bilateral hydronephrosis. What is the most likely explanation for these findings?

A) Prune Belly syndrome
B) Esophageal atresia
C) Premature rupture of membranes
D) Posterior urethral valves
E) Both A and D

384) Each of the following is a part of the treatment of congenital nephrotic syndrome *except:*

A) ACE inhibitors
B) Corticosteroids
C) High protein diet
D) Thyroxine
E) Low dose aspirin

385) You are caring for a teenager with elevated blood pressure on 3 separate occasions by 3 different nurses. Which of the following would be the most appropriate initial steps in managing this patient?

A) Lasix
B) Atenolol
C) Repeat the blood pressure in a week
D) Nutrition and exercise consultation
E) Reassurance that hypertension will resolve

Rheumatology

386) All of the following are appropriate for preventing recurrences of rheumatic fever *EXCEPT* for:

A) Benzathine penicillin G IM
B) Penicillin V PO
C) Cefaclor PO
D) Erythromycin PO
E) Sulfadiazine

387) A child who is new to your practice comes in for his first appointment. He has been diagnosed in the past with acute rheumatic fever. The mom brings in an 8-foot high pile of downloaded printouts, miraculously, the forklift and pallets leave only 2 or 3 scratches in your paneling so you tip the forklift operator handsomely.

She wants know the primary *long-term* concerns she should have about her son. You tell her:

A) Permanent joint damage caused by the migratory polyarthritis
B) The effects of mitral valve insufficiency
C) Aortic insufficiency leading to heart failure.
D) Chronic pain secondary to the subcutaneous nodules
E) The marginal lifestyle of those exhibiting erythema marginatum.

388) The <u>earliest</u> sign of Kawasaki disease is:

A) Strawberry daiquiri tongue
B) An obsessive desire to drive a motorcycle
C) High persistent fever for well over a week's duration
D) Non-purulent conjunctivitis
E) Peeling skin on hands and feet

389) Each of the following is among the major Jones criteria for diagnosing rheumatic fever with the *EXCEPTION* of:

A) Migratory arthritis
B) Carditis
C) Erythema marginatum
D) Erythema infectiosum
E) Subcutaneous nodules

390) Match each number (synovial fluid description) to its diagnosis on the right

1) Clear, WBC < 200
2) Clear, WBC < 2000, increased viscosity
3) Cloudy, 5000 WBC, decreased viscosity
4) Cloudy, 20,000 WBC, decreased viscosity
5) Yellow, 200,000 decreased viscosity
6) Yellow, bouquet with a kick and a slight after-taste, 10,000 + epithelial cells

(A) Kendall Jackson Chardonnay
(B) JRA
(C) Normal joint fluid aspirate
(D) Rheumatic fever
(E) Septic arthritis
(F) Trauma

391) Match the numbered condition on the left with the lettered indicator or causative factor on the right.

1) Mixed connective tissue disease
2) Antiphospholipid syndrome
3) Wegener's granulomatosis
4) Schönlein-Henoch purpura
5) Systemic lupus erythematosus

(A) False-positive VDRL
(B) Systemic vasculitis
(C) IgA nephropathy
(D) Antibodies to Smith antigen (anti-SM)
(E) High titers of antibodies to an RNase-sensitive component of extractable nuclear antigen

392) The vast majority of children with hypermobility syndrome[11] will:

A) Need a cardiac evaluation to evaluate for mitral prolapse, aneurysms, and aortic dissection common with connective tissue disorders

B) Need a complete ophthalmological workup to rule out lens dislocation and iritis

C) Never come to your attention at all

D) Require extensive genetic and metabolic workup

E) Be well known to the lobby security guard[12] and your office staff because of their "cocktail party personality" and playful demeanor

393) Each of the following is a hematological manifestation of systemic lupus erythematosus *except* for:

A) Anemia of chronic illness

B) Hemolytic anemia

C) Thrombocytopenia

D) Leukocytosis

E) Leukopenia

394) Which one of the following manifestations of neonatal lupus erythematosus is irreversible?

A) Thrombocytopenia

B) Congenital heart block

C) Cutaneous lupus lesions

D) Hepatitis

E) Hepatomegaly

395) Each of the following medications is used to treat various manifestations of lupus *except for:*

A) Non steroidal anti inflammatory medications

B) Glucocorticosteroid

C) Insulin

D) Sunscreen

E) Cyclophosphamide

---

[11] Double-jointed, as it is commonly known on playgrounds.

[12] The one with the pencil-thin mustache and odd-smelling cologne.

Substance Abuse

396) The most widely used drug among teenagers is:

A) PCP
B) Ecstasy
C) Alcohol
D) Marijuana
E) Love

397) You are evaluating a 16 year old boy in the ER who returned home late from a party. He is very anxious, restless and animated. He is complaining of abdominal cramping. On physical examination you note mydriasis tachycardia, mild hypertension and increased deep tendon reflexes.

Which of the following would explain the patient's behavior?

A) Undiagnosed bipolar disease
B) Amphetamine abuse
C) PCP abuse
D) Alcohol toxicity
E) Cannabis abuse

398) You are evaluating a 15 year old boy who reportedly had been smoking marijuana possibly laced with PCP. On physical exam he is disoriented and stares blankly. His muscles are rigid. He is slightly tachycardic with elevated blood pressure. The most appropriate next step in managing this patient would be:

A) Place patient in a windowless secure room
B) Provide rectal Valium
C) Measure serum myoglobin
D) Naloxone intramuscular
E) Acidification of urine

399) Which of the following is true regarding drug use in the United States?

A) Drug use among high school students was at its highest in the 1980's
B) Cigarette smoking among 8th-12 graders has increased over the past decade
C) The use of performance enhancing drugs decreases the likelihood of use of other illicit drugs
D) Homosexual adolescents have rates of substance abuse that are significantly higher than heterosexual peers
E) Inhalant abuse is more prevalent among 12th graders than 8th graders

400) You are asked to medically clear a teenage boy for a psychiatric evaluation. Over the past few weeks he has had violent outbursts and has exhibited hypomania.

His blood pressure is 125/85 is built like a football player. You note on physical exam the presence of acne, primarily pustular –papular as well as bilateral gynecomastia. His voice is higher pitched than would be expected for his Tanner stage.

The abuse of which of the following substances is the likely explanation?

A) The refrigerator
B) Marijuana
C) Methylphenidate
D) Anabolic steroids
E) Growth hormone

Answers

Adolescent

1)   D)   Rapid refeeding of patients who are severely malnourished (which somebody who is 35% below ideal weight would be) can result in hypophosphatemia. leading to potential cardiac failure, coma, and hemolytic anemia.

2)   C)   Factors associated with early initiation of early initiation of sexual activity include, early onset of puberty, sexual abuse, and lower socioeconomic status. Factors which associated with a later initiation of sexual activity include parental consistency, firmness in discipline at home and high academic achievement.

Access to condoms in school based clinics increased the use of condoms with intercourse but does not impact the rates of sexual activity or early initiation of sexual activity.

3)   B)   For every adolescent killed in a motor vehicle accident 100 non fatal injuries occur many leading to permanent disability and is therefore a leading cause of both morbidity and mortality in teenagers.

A 16 year old is 20 times more likely to have crash while driving than the general population and they also have a low use of seat belts while driving. While adolescents feel immortal they clearly are not.

4)   D)   Adolescents have a limited ability to link cause and effect when it comes to high risk or unhealthy behavior including, seat belt use, overeating, smoking, and drug use. Often this behavior is a way of differentiating from their parent and obtaining a self identity. Therefore signing a contract with their parents will likely have an opposite effect. However adolescents do care a lot about their physical appearance and their physical performance. Therefore emphasizing the impact smoking will have on their athletic performance will likely had an impact in your attempts to get them to stop smoking.

5) D) Approximately 30% of gay youths have attempted suicide at least once; therefore depression and suicide ideation are not rare among homosexual teenagers. Transient homosexual experimentation is *not uncommon* in teenagers. Adolescents who are emotionally attracted to members of the same gender usually do *not* engage in sexual activity.

6) D) Scoliosis inheritance is multifactorial not x-linked. It is more common in girls than boys and is defined as a curvature of the spine greater than 10 degrees. Adolescent idiopathic scoliosis is defined as scoliosis whose onset is seen in children older than 10.

Mild-moderate pulmonary compromise can be seen in spin curvature greater than 60 degrees.

7) C) 25 % of sexually active adolescents become infected with sexually transmitted diseases each year. *Chlamydia trachomatis* and *Neisseria gonorrhea* can be asymptomatic in both males and females, and it is now possible to diagnose both through urine "amplification" techniques. These techniques are less invasive and should result in increased compliance and willingness to be tested.

8) A) Urine sampling is both more sensitive (less false negatives) and more specific (less false positives) than culture. However, when needed for forensic purposes i.e. where sexual abuse or assault is a consideration, cultures are still needed as definitive evidence.

In contrast to UTI, the urine sample for sexually transmitted diseases testing needs to be from the beginning of the stream rather than the mid stream and the perineum *should not be cleaned first*. Therefore, one urine sample cannot be used for both tests.

Thus it is very difficult to obtain both samples with "one sitting". If you think about it, one would have to first collect urine for the sexually transmitted diseases sample, "suspend" the stream while cleaning the perineum, and then collect for the UTI. This would require Olympic-level skills, and the second sample would probably not be very reliable.

9)   A)   *Hyper*thyroidism, *hypo*thyroidism, hyperprolactinemia and ovarian failure can all result in anovulatory uterine bleeding. Cystic fibrosis would not be a significant consideration in the differential diagnosis.

10)   C)   The patient in the vignette is presenting with cyclical abnormal bleeding which is by definition, *menorrhagia*. Given the strong family history for the same, this is suggestive of a bleeding disorder. Of the 3 bleeding disorders listed, von Willebrand disease is the only one that makes sense. Factor VIII and IX are X-linked and primarily affect males.

There is nothing to suggest polycystic ovary syndrome or Crohn's disease.

Allergy & Immunology

11)   1)   C
        2)   D
        3)   A
        4)   B

An Arthus/ Immune complex reaction is a Type 3 allergic reaction

A delayed hypersensitivity reaction such as contact dermatitis is a Type 4 reaction

An anaphylactoid reaction would be a Type 1 allergic reaction

A Type 2 allergic reaction is antibody mediated

12)   D)   Common variable immunodeficiency can result in both defects in cell mediated immunity and hypoglobulinemia. Patients will present with recurrent respiratory problems and occasionally vague GI symptoms and anemia. A poor response to the vaccine wouldn't explain the recurrent respiratory symptoms. X-linked severe immunodeficiency would have a much more (as the name implies) severe picture and HIV would not likely present with a thriving child with a negative physical examination, especially on the Boards.

13)   A)   Predisposing factors to food allergy include a positive family history of atopic disease, early antigen exposure during the first few days of life, and *low* (rather than high) IgA in mother's colostrum.

IgE mediated reactions are felt to play a major role, and food proteins found in breast milk can serve as milk allergens.

14)   E)   Since they note that the baby is being exclusively breast fed, the rash is probably related to this. The description is of atopic dermatitis. It is very possible that something in the mother's diet is responsible and the allergen is crossing over into the breast milk, causing a reaction in the infant. Skin testing the mother will not be of help since she is not the one with the rash.

Skin testing the infant will not be helpful due to the fact that the rash is diffuse and the infant has been given diphenhydramine.

The antihistamine will interfere with the accuracy of the skin testing. The presence of IgE in the infant to various allergens will help determine the cause. Switching to soy formula may not be of help since the infant may have been sensitized to soy formula as well.

15)   C)   IgA deficiency is the most common primary immunodeficiency. Since this is the antibody found in mucosal linings, it results in frequent infections of the respiratory, GI, and urogenital tracts.

16)   E)   Thymic transplantation is most successful in patients with complete DiGeorge syndrome who have a significant T-lymphocyte deficiency.

17)   E)   B cells in patients with x-linked hyper IgM syndrome can make IgM but cannot make IgG, IGA or IgE. Therefore IgM levels are high and IgG, IgA, and IgE levels are low.

Treatment with intravenous gammaglobulin is indicated. In addition these patients are at increased risk for infection with P. jiroveci and prophylaxis is indicated.

18)   D)   IgA deficiency is the *most* common primary immunodeficiency. Most patients with this disorder are actually asymptomatic.

Symptomatic cases usually also have defects in one or more IgG subclasses.

IgA deficiency is *not* an indication for replacement immunoglobulin therapy.

Patients with IgA deficiency often have circulating anti-IgA antibody. Even though most commercial IgG preparations contain negligible amounts of IgA, even this small amount can cause an anaphylactoid reaction in patients with IgA deficiency.

This fact is often tested on the boards.

19)   C)   Growth velocity is reduced during the first year of treatment. However catchup growth after the first year results in the achievement of adult height.

Acne, mood swings and weight gain do occur although not as frequently as is seen with systemic steroid use.

Oral candidiasis is one of the more common complications reduced with mouth rinsing after inhalation.

20) E) Topical diphenhydramine would likely irritate the skin and topical hydrocortisone would have no long term role intreating chronic urticaria

Hydroxyzine and diphenhydramine can be sedating making them poor candidates for long term treatment.

Fexofenadine is a 2nd generation non sedating H1 antihistamine and would be the most appropriate long term treatment for chronic urticaria of those listed.

Cardiology

21) D) The 4 components of Tetralogy of Fallot include:
1) Pulmonary stenosis
2) Right ventricular hypertrophy
3) Overriding aorta
4) VSD

Tricuspid atresia is not part of the tetralogy of Fallot.

22)
1) E - Ventricular Fibrillation. This is the classic, disorganized nonfunctional heartbeat.
2) F - Ventricular Tachycardia.
3) G - Wolf Parkinson White syndrome. There is a short PR interval making for the classic "Delta wave." (Yes, the other Delta wave is what you see on a balcony during Mardi gras, usually after a few drinks.)
4) A - Sinus arrhythmia. This is due to an inconsistent rate of impulse coming from the sinus node.
5) C - 2nd degree AV block. Here there is a prolonged PR interval followed by dropped ventricular beats.
6) D - 3rd degree AV block. Here no impulses get through to the ventricle.
7) H - Premature ventricular contraction.
8) B - Supraventricular tachycardia.

23)   1) D
          2) E
          3) G
          4) A
          5) F
          6) C
          7) H
          8) B

The murmur heard in **pulmonary stenosis** is distinguished from aortic stenosis and Still's murmur by the presence of an **ejection click that varies with respiration.**

Aortic stenosis is associated with a **systolic ejection click that does <u>not</u> vary with respiration.**

With **coarctation of the aorta, a continuous murmur over the back can be heard with long-standing disease and development of collateral flow.**

The classic murmur heard with an **atrial septal defect** is the **abnormal fixed splitting of S2.**

The murmur of **mitral insufficiency** is **holosystolic, heard best at the apex.** The murmur can *radiate to the axillae and the back* and can mimic the murmur of a ventricular septal defect.

24)   C) Disorders causing cyanotic heart disease begin with a T, but do not expect a fastball down the middle. Thus, d-Transposition and anomalous (total) pulmonary venous return both start with a T. However they may not make it that obvious on the exam.

In order to take advantage of this mnemonic you must change d-Transposition to plain old transposition of the great arteries. Anomalous (total) pulmonary venous return must be changed the more familiar Total anomalous pulmonary venous return.

Aortic insufficiency is not associated with cyanotic heart disease it does not start with a T no matter how you manipulate it.

25)   C)   A medium-pitched, vibratory or "musical", relatively short, systolic ejection murmur that is heard best along the left lower and midsternal border is a description of the most common innocent murmur.

26)   E)   A **left axis deviation** can be seen with
· AV canal defects
· Tricuspid atresia,
· Double outlet right ventricle,
· Normal heart (sometimes)

With a hypertrophic cardiomyopathy, one would have an increased left ventricular mass; however, *one would not expect to see a left axis deviation on EKG.*

27)   A)   This child is *acyanotic*, so the diagnosis won't be one of the cyanotic heart diseases, which begin with a "T" (ruling out tetralogy of Fallot and transposition of the great vessels).

This narrows us down to two choices ASD and VSD.

The clinical scenario including the murmur is most consistent with an infant with a large VSD that is going into heart failure.

28)   B)   **It is the increased arterial PO2 that is largely responsible for the closing of the patent ductus arteriosus (PDA).**

Additional factors include the decreased pulmonary vascular resistance and decreased circulating prostaglandin level.

Regardless, it is the increased PO2 that is the key player.

29)   D)   The gold standard for diagnosing subacute bacterial endocarditis would be a blood culture. This is an example where it is important to focus on what is being asked (also called "reading the question") and not jumps to instinct in picking 24-hour EKG.

Echocardiogram, although not one of the choices, would also *not be the best answer*. Although it may identify vegetations, this in and of itself would not rule out bacterial endocarditis.

Had the question been phrased differently—asking the most diagnostic *cardiac* study—then cardiac echo would be the correct answer. Always read the question and circle the key words so they stand out.

30)   C)   Truncus arteriosus is characterized by a large ventricular septal defect over which a large, single great vessel (truncus) arises. This single great vessel carries blood both to the body and to the lungs.

Therefore the pulmonary artery and the aorta combine for one vessel with partially saturated blood and equal pressure. Since both ventricles are essentially contiguous you have the same pressure and saturation seen in the truncus (combined vessel)

The pulmonary vein and left atrium are largely unaffected and their pressure and saturation is the same as you would see in a normal heart.

The key to answering this correctly is the same pressures and saturations in the common truncus, RV and LV.

31)   B)   The key to answering this question correctly is to focus on the variation from the normal heart.

You have an increased pressure in the right ventricle consistent with pulmonary stenosis and right ventricular hypertrophy. In addition the LV and RV oxygen saturation are equal due to the VSD. This is consistent with tetralogy of Fallot.

32)   C)   This cardiac catheterization demonstrates

· Increased saturations on the right side of the heart equal to the left (which is less than normal)

· Increased pressure in all chambers and gradients on the right side and decreased pressure in all chambers and gradients on the left side.

This is consistent with total anomalous pulmonary venous return where none of the four veins that drain blood from the lungs to the heart is attached to the left atrium. In TAPVR, oxygenated blood returns to the right atrium instead.

33)   C)   In addition to coronary aneurysms cardiac complications also include myocarditis and valvulitis. High dose aspirin is used during the acute phase until fever subsides.

Following this low dose aspirin is continued for several weeks or until the platelet count returns to normal.

Coronary aneurysms start developing early in the disease but they do not manifest until later. Therefore cardiac echo done at the time of diagnosis is to assess for myocarditis which may not have manifested clinically yet.

IV gamma globulin is given during the acute phase

34)   C)   The history and presentation of this patient is consistent with costochondritis. Their noting that the grandfather died of an MI at 65 and the father is being treated for hypertension are decoys. Cardiac disease in relatives older than 55 would not reflect a risk for cardiac disease in a young person. There is no evidence for GERD causing the chest pain.

There is no evidence of abdominal pain since the physical exam is benign. The unremarkable physical exam does not rule out costochondritis either. It might have resolved by the time the patient got to the doctor's office.

35)   C)   The most appropriate first step would be to measure serum triglycerides and cholesterol before moving on to any therapeutic modalities.

Cardiac echo and stress test would be premature at this point.

Cognition, Language & Learning

36) E) Most learning disabilities are life long and therefore continue into adulthood. Learning disabilities, which are very specific, do not reflect IQ and can therefore coexist with an above average IQ.

Learning disabilities are diagnosed based on history and neuro-psychometric testing.

However, if they ask you for the most helpful part of any evaluation for a learning disorder, the answer is *history*.

37) D) Difficulties with organizational skills would be associated with ADD but would not, in and of itself, represent a specific learning disability.

The others—the three R's of Reading, 'Riting and 'Rithmatic, and dyslexia (whoops! Make that two R's and a D) —would represent specific learning disabilities. That reminds me of my favorite dyslexia joke: did you hear about the agnostic, dyslexic, insomniac? Yeah, he was up all night wondering if there was a D-O-G.

38) B) A child who can walk upstairs with one hand being held, can turn the pages of a textbook 3 pages at a time, can speak 10 words and can identify 1 body part is either an 18 month old child or a pediatrician who just completed 2 days of answering board questions and is headed home.

39)   D)   Children younger than 6 years *suspected* of having mental retardation would be more appropriately characterized as having *"global developmental disorder"*

One exception would be in the context of a diagnosed recognizable syndrome associated with mental retardation where a mental retardation would be the appropriate characterization

Close to **50%** of children with *severe* mental retardation have **behavioral problems**.

Approximately **50%** of children with cerebral palsy will have some degree of mental retardation.

Seizure disorders are approximately **10 times** more common in children who have mental retardation

The prevalence of sleep disorders is **inversely proportional** to **intelligence.**

40)   C)   Infants diagnosed with a syndrome known to be associated with mental retardation become eligible at birth

Children diagnosed prior to their 3rd birthday should be referred to EIP as soon as the local board of education will accept referral.

Critical Care

41)   D)   With the exception of hypoglycemia, all of the factors listed can interfere with an accurate reading. Hypoglycemia can result in tachypnea but this should not impair oxygen saturation readings.

Carboxyhemoglobin absorbs the same amount of light as oxyhemoglobin therefore the combination is read as if it is oxygen and the reading is falsely elevated.

At high levels of methemoglobinemia the pulse oximeter reads a saturation of 85%, regardless of the true percentage of oxyhemoglobin therefore interfering with the accuracy.

42) 1) C
    2) E
    3) G
    4) A
    5) H
    6) F
    7) D
    8) B

This is another board "grid" classic and bound to be on your exam. It should be an easy lay-up. It is best to take a systematic approach to this question. *Even though they say you can use each answer more than once this is rarely the case and you are best advised to cross out the answers as you select them.*

Respiratory acidosis, since you are dealing with acidosis, first look for a low pH, bicarb will be high in an attempt to compensate but not fully compensated, thus the low pH.

Respiratory acidosis (compensated) will have similar numbers as uncompensated with a pH close to normal.

Respiratory alkalosis will have a high pH and a low CO_2 along with insufficient compensatory low bicarb that has not impacted pH.

Respiratory alkalosis (compensated) pH will be high, with a low CO_2 and low enough bicarb to bring the pH close to normal.

The same applies to the metabolic form of acidosis and alkalosis with the compensated forms having a pH close to normal.

With the combined disorders you have contributions from CO_2 and bicarb pulling the pH in the same direction.

43)   C)   The fact that a child is stable in the ED is not the deciding factor regarding discharge and observation at home. Of the choices listed the only scenario where a child can be safely discharged home and observed is with a child submerged less than one minute not requiring CPR.

A child requiring CPR, aspirated water, had a seizure, or a change of mental status in the field, could deteriorate and needs to be observed in the hospital for at least 24 hours. Tachypnea could be a sign that acute respiratory distress syndrome and/or aspiration pneumonia could be developing.

44)   D)   In the past *hyperventilation syndrome* was felt to be synonymous with *panic attack.* However hyperventilation can be triggered by other factors including change in position from laying down to standing. This would suggest increased baroreceptor sensitivity may be the cause in these situations not anxiety.

Hyperventilation syndrome is breathing in excess of metabolic requirements resulting in *hypo*capnia rather than *hypercapnia.*

It is very easy to see hypo and hyper as the same in the heat of the battle so pay particular attention to this when reading the questions *carefully.*

45)   E)   The clinical scenario is consistent with a diagnosis of meningococcemia. While ceftriaxone alone would be sufficient to treat this patient, you must also cover for the possibility of penicillin and cephalosporin resistant pneumococcus, Staph aureus, and enterococcus. Therefore the correct treatment would be IV Vancomycin *and* Ceftriaxone.

46)   E)   Polyomavirus hominis (BKV) infection is an important cause of late onset kidney graft rejection.

Dermatology

47)   1)   (D) - Tinea capitis
         2)   (E) - Alopecia areata
         3)   (C) - Trichotillomania
         4)   (B) - Alopecia totalis
         5)   (A) - Alopecia neurotica.

On the exam tinea capitis will often be described as scalp inflammation and **black dots.**

Alopecia areata will be described as complete areas of smooth hair loss with no inflammation or discoloration.

Trichotillomania is incomplete patches of hair loss with hair shafts of varying lengths.

Alopecia totalis as the name implies, means "total baldness" in Latin. Therefore even the eyebrows are involved.

Alopecia neurotica is baldness as a result of being totally neurotic and hyper such as a pediatrician going from a total head of hair to total baldness while preparing for the boards. This is also known as "Board Baldness".

48)   E)   This is a classic description of tinea pedis, or "athlete's foot". The fact that the sibling has it is a red herring set to throw you off the trail toward thinking the diagnosis is scabies. However there is nothing else in the history to suggest this.

Hyperhidrosis[1] would explain the foul odor but not the other physical findings described. Tinea pedis in and of itself does not result in a foul odor. However, a moist environment in the shoes would lead to a foul odor akin to a damp basement in the summertime.

49)   E)   Erythema infectiosum, which is the rash associated with fifth disease, can be described as a "slapped cheek" appearance along with a reticular rash on the extremities. Human parvovirus B19 is felt to be the etiological agent.

---

[1] Excessive sweating of the palms and soles in response to emotional stimuli.

50)   F)   *Neisseria meningitidis* bacteremia may result in the release of an endotoxin, which can lead to DIC and deplete clotting factors and protein C. This is especially problematic in kids already deficient in Protein C.

Deficiency of protein C can lead to cutaneous infarctions called *purpura fulminans,* which is an ominous sign.

51)   F)   The rash described is "erythema nodosum". It is a hypersensitivity reaction that can be associated with any of the conditions listed. However, they asked for the **most likely** cause, and that would be Group A *Strep.*

52)   E)   In cases initially thought to be *severe seborrheic dermatitis* that do not resolve and progress to ulcerated lesions coupled with petechiae and purpura, histiocytosis X must be ruled out. This is best accomplished by skin biopsy.

53)   E)   The rash is a typical description of Gianotti-Crosti syndrome. It is often associated with viral infections, including EBV, hepatitis B, and CMV, among others.

If you picked erythema erythema you would be red red in the face with embarrassment.

54)   A)   Baseline laboratory studies are not necessary when griseofulvin is given to children. Topical antifungal agents are not effective because the fungus of tinea capitis resides within the hair shafts, *not on them.* However, topical steroids can sometimes help alleviate the inflammatory reaction seen with tinea capitis. For better absorption, it is recommended that griseofulvin be taken with lipid-containing foods.

55) C) With no papules or pustules, the treatment is aimed toward taking care of the comedones.[2] Since retinoic acid[3] is the single most effective agent in the treatment of comedonial acne, it is the correct answer. The results of retinoic acid are not seen for 3-6 months and sunscreen must be used with retinoic acid because of the increased sensitivity to sunlight. Turn out the light while waiting.

56) E) Kwashiorkor often results in eczematous changes along with hypopigmentation and dry skin.

Endocrinology

57) B) The newborn screen for hypothyroid measures TSH levels. A positive screen needs to be confirmed by measuring a serum TSH level. However treatment should be started before the results are confirmed. Serum free T4 could be done but this is not the most appropriate next step in confirming the screen.

58) E) Children who develop hypothyroidism after 3 years of age won't develop *permanent* impairment of intellectual or neurological function. In this case it is important to read the question carefully. There can be impairment but it is reversible with treatment, therefore the italicized word *permanent* is important here.

59) A) A delay in the diagnosis and implementation of treatment with thyroxine after 3 months of age carries an increased risk of impaired intellectual function and neuropsychological development.

---

[2] Dilated epithelial lined follicular sac filled with keratinous material, lipid, and bacteria; much easier to just say comedones.
[3] Tretinoin = Retin-A®

60)   C)   The most appropriate treatment for idiopathic central precocious puberty is leuprolide which is GnRH agonist. This works by down regulating the GnRH and suspending premature pubertal development.

61)   C)   The combination of a drop-off in height, maintenance of weight and pubertal delay points to hypothyroidism, Cushing disease or growth hormone deficiency.

With familial short stature one would expect to see low percentile for height and weight maintained from birth to adulthood. In constitutional growth delay one would expect bone age below chronological age however one would not expect a drop-off in the height curve.

In Crohn disease and nutritional deficiency one would not expect to see maintenance of weight in the 50th percentile.

Their mentioning that the other sibling was a slow grower is a red herring.

62)   D)   Erythrocyte sedimentation rate

The combination of drop-off in both weight and height points to a gastrointestinal disorder such as Crohn disease. Therefore of the choices listed the most appropriate initial screen would be an erythrocyte sedimentation rate.

63)   D)   Of the choices listed the best screen for growth hormone deficiency would be IGF-1 which stands for "Insulin like growth factor – 1". Another correct choice if it were listed is "Insulin like growth factor binding protein – 3".

64)   D)   If you suspect a diagnosis of celiac disease in a child and have documented normal IgA concentrations the most appropriate initial screen would be tissue transglutaminase antibody level.

65) D) The history is consistent with delayed puberty due to a central nervous system cause most likely a pituitary tumor. Of all the choices the most appropriate study to order would be a serum prolactin level which would be elevated with a pituitary tumor. [4]

66) A) If you simply divide the parents' height in inches by 12 you discover that they are both around 5 feet tall. Clearly this boy will not be playing center in the NBA all-star game. Thus, the diagnosis is genetic short stature and "normal". The only pattern that makes sense, therefore, would be choice A.

67) A) Subcutaneous calcification does occur in hypoparathyroidism. In hypoparathyroidism one would expect to see low serum calcium levels. Hematuria sometimes occurs with *hypercalcemia.* Therefore, hematuria would not be expected in hypoparathyroidism, nor would hypertension or hypoglycemia. Mucocutaneous candidiasis can occur, and when it does it *precedes* the development of hypoparathyroidism. It is also not "frequently" associated with the diagnosis. *Again, read the key words in the last sentence of the question.*

68) E) The combination or normal Vitamin D 1, 25, Vitamin D, 25, Serum Calcium and parathyroid hormone along with elevated alkaline phosphatase and low serum phosphate in a child with clinical rickets is consistent with a diagnosis of familial hypophosphatemic rickets.

69) A) By noting that the infant is African American and lactose intolerant they are steering you toward a diagnosis of Vitamin D deficient rickets. There are two risk factors at play here. One risk factor is dark skin resulting in decreased exposure to ultraviolet light. Another is lactose intolerance which could result in decreased dairy product and Vitamin D intake.

The elevated PTH and alkaline phosphatase coupled with the decreased calcium, phosphate and Vitamin D, 25 confirms the correct diagnosis.

Hypophosphatasia is an inherited disorder of poor alkaline phosphatase production and not consistent with the clinical scenario in the question.

---

[4] If you must no why this is because of pressure on the pituitary stalk resulting in disruption of dopaminergic inhibition of prolactin. Elevated prolactin levels would interfere with normal menstrual cycles and pubertal. Now get back to work on material you might actually be tested on!

70)   B)   Vitamin D dependent rickets Type 1 is due to impaired production of Vitamin D 1, 25 by the kidney. This results in very low levels of Vitamin D1, 25 and no improvement with Vitamin D replacement as one would expect with Vitamin D deficient rickets.

71)   C)   Vitamin D dependent rickets Type 2 is due to end organ resistance to Vitamin D. Therefore the primary way to differentiate Type 1 from Type 2 is the Vitamin D 1, 25 levels which are elevated in Type 2 and decreased in Type 1.

72)   B)   Metabolic syndrome has some overlap with type 2 diabetes but it is not the same. There is some overlap but it is a different entity. However the important points to know are:

The International Diabetes foundation established the following criteria:

- Fasting triglycerides greater than 150
- High density lipoprotein cholesterol less than 40
- Blood pressure greater than 130/85
- Fasting glucose greater than 100 OR previously diagnosed with diabetes type 2

Acanthosis nigricans seen in diabetes type 2 is not a criterion for metabolic syndrome and neither is family history of diabetes type 2 disease.

73)   E)   When presented with unexplained deterioration or recurrent deterioration of a chronic condition in an adolescent, *poor compliance* should always be a consideration. This is the most likely explanation for the recurrent episodes of DKA in this otherwise appropriately managed teenager. The question notes that the patient is "on an appropriate insulin regimen" and the nutritionist has "set up" an appropriate diet. This does not mean the patient is compliant. If the patient was compliant this would have been specifically stated. Once again read the question carefully.

The Somogyi effect is is caused by nighttime hypoglycemia, which leads to a rebound hyperglycemia in the early morning hours.

The Dawn effect also presents as morning hyperglycemia. However it is not related to nocturnal hyperglycemia.

74)   E)   The younger the child is at the age of onset, the more likely they have Type 1 diabetes. However, in adolescence this is a less important factor. Type 1 diabetes, in addition to being an autoimmune phenomenon, can also be "idiopathic".[5]

Type 2 is due to insulin resistance and some secretory deficits. While Type 2 disease is seen 'primarily' in obese children, if you assume a lean child cannot have Type 2 disease, you may misdiagnose and incorrectly manage the child.

75)   1)   (B)
2)   (B)
3)   (B)
4)   (A)
5)   (C)
6)   (D)

An *incidental diagnosis* of Type 2 disease is in an otherwise asymptomatic patient is common. On the other hand Type 1 usually presents with notable symptoms. Type 2 can present with a vaginal monilial infection. Acanthosis nigricans is a hyperpigmentation noted in the skin folds of the neck and flexion areas. It is associated with Type 2 diabetes as well as obesity in which there are chronically elevated insulin levels due to insulin resistance. However, any obese patient should be evaluated for Type 2 diabetes.

One would only expect to see autoantibodies in Type 1 disease. Stress can exacerbate both Type 1 and Type 2 disease.

Arcaneis testus is Latin (or maybe Greek) for "arcane test", which is what the board exam is. It is believed that the current system utilizing number two pencils and dots was actually used by Hippocrates when he "sat" for the boards.[6]

---

[5] Which is Latin for "We have no idea?"
[6] He also served as his own proctor the second time he took the exam.

76)   C)   With the exception of the occasional red herring, there is a reason you are given each bit of information, including **the fact that the mother is a Type 1 diabetic**. **They do not mention that the child is diabetic and this is important** *Type 1 diabetes is not known to have a genetic link, so any disturbance in glucose metabolism is probably not biological.*

The source of the insulin is either endogenous or exogenous (i.e., in the cases involving Münchhausen by proxy). *The C-peptide levels correlate with the endogenously produced insulin. A high insulin level combined with a low C-peptide level indicates factitious hypoglycemia* and would implicate the mother. Nice work Dr. Gregory House! This would prove that the mother is administering exogenous insulin to the child, resulting in episodes of hypoglycemia and confirming a diagnosis of Münchhausen by proxy.

77)   1) (C)
2) (B)
3) (C)
4) (D)
5) (D)
6) (B)
7) (B)

Hashimoto's thyroiditis is also known as chronic lymphocytic thyroiditis and can result in *hyper*thyroidism (hashitoxicosis) or *hypo*thyroidism. Both Graves' and Hashimoto's are triggered by components of the immune system Hashimoto's by lymphocytic infiltration and Graves' by human thyroid stimulating hormone (which is an IgG). Neither one represents precancerous lesions. The owner of the diner on *Happy Days* was Arnold and, although he is of Japanese ancestry (and later starred in *The Karate Kid*); the actor is Noriyuki "Pat" Morita, not Hashimoto.

Patients are with Hashimoto's disease can be clinically euthyroid or hypothyroid. Most are **asymptomatic** and are discovered by the presence of a goiter. In such cases T4 and TSH should be checked regularly.

ENT

78)   C)   No effect at all. Expectorants have an effect by thinning out secretions under experimental conditons but not under clinical conditions. Since this is the clinical not the experimental boards, C is the answer.

79)   C)   All lymphoid tissue reaches maximum size between 5 to 7 years. This may be asked straight out or in the form of a graph where you will have to compare with the growth of other tissue.

80)   1) (B)
          2) (C)
          3) (A)

Laryngomalacia would be described as wet *inspiratory* stridor.

Paralyzed vocal cords would present as high pitched inspiratory stridor.

Tracheomalacia would be described as *expiratory stridor.*

81)   C)   **A bark-like cough coupled with inspiratory stridor is typical of viral croup.** In addition, subglottic narrowing is the typical "steeple sign" seen on x-ray with viral croup. Epiglottitis is unlikely given the age of the child and their not describing fever or severe respiratory distress typical of epiglottitis.

82)   A)   The scenario described is of **peritonsillar abscess,** which is typically **unilateral,** not bilateral. Peritonsillar abscess can be preceded by pharyngitis. Parenteral antibiotics should be chosen to cover group B strep as well as anaerobes. Penicillin would be the drug of choice. Trismus[7] is a common tip that the diagnosis is peritonsillar abscess.

---

[7] Whatever that is. Wither way Merry Trismus!

83) E) In a child of this age group, **unilateral foul-smelling nasal discharge** would be most consistent with a **foreign body.** There is no mention of the child being febrile, making sinusitis unlikely; besides, it would typically be bilateral, as would allergic rhinitis. Unilateral choanal atresia would present with non-purulent discharge. Juvenile angiofibroma would present with nose bleeding.

84) A) The combination of swelling over the postauricular area with outward and downward displacement of the pinna is virtually diagnostic for mastoiditis. Without any evidence of discharge, a *cholesteatoma* is unlikely, as are any of the other choices presented.

85) E) **The only "absolute" indication for tonsillectomy is obstructive sleep apnea.** Any other indication would be considered controversial. While snoring audible enough to cross state lines would hamper ones social or married life, it would not be an indication for surgery, and neither would any acute or chronic infection. Some ENT surgeons would recommend tonsillectomy in the face of 7 episodes of tonsillitis in a year, but it would not be considered an absolute indication for purposes of the exam.

86) B) The *most likely* cause of a "sudden onset" of bilateral sensorineural deafness would be *viral labyrinthitis.* **In general, if something is of an acute onset and you had no idea of the answer, then a viral etiology would not be a bad choice.** The degree of severity and/or recovery is variable.

Autoimmune disorders are typically gradual in onset, and hearing loss due to drug toxicity would be gradual as well. The chances of a foreign body causing bilateral deafness would be unusual, especially when they are confirming that it is sensorineural.

87)   E)   Tympanometry measures tympanic membrane (TM) compliance and middle ear pressure. In most cases an immobile eardrum is caused by fluid in the middle ear. However, tympanometry in and of itself could not be used to diagnose otitis externa, otitis media, or the source of the middle ear effusion causing the decreased compliance. It also could not identify hearing loss, and certainly could not distinguish the type of hearing loss (conductive vs. sensorineural).

          It only helps establish impaired mobility of the tympanic membrane which should be used with other clinical findings in establishing a diagnosis.

88)   B)   This would be an example of **subhyoid ectopic thyroid** tissue, and it may be the only thyroid tissue she has. Therefore, it should not be removed. Since her height and weight would point toward hypothyroidism, it would be prudent to obtain thyroid hormone levels as the first step. Ectopic thyroid tissue may produce adequate thyroid hormone for several years and then fail in early childhood, which is probably the case in this scenario.

          Therefore radionuclide thyroid scan would be appropriate to identify if this mass represents the only thyroid tissue this patient has.

          Keep this in mind when shown a mass at the base of the tongue. **You must distinguish it from a ranula based on the clinical scenario...**

89)   C)   Penicillin remains the champion antibiotic to use for dental infections.

90)   D)   The most appropriate intervention in this setting would be to discontinue bottle feeding at night as well as nocturnal breast feeding. Both have been linked to development of dental caries in both age groups

91)   A)   Hearing loss is the most common complication of otitis media. It is not clear if tympanostomy tubes help prevent hearing loss in chronic otitis.

92) D) The symptoms are consistent with a sinus infection. However the chronicity of symptoms makes for a diagnosis of chronic rather than acute sinusitis.

93) D) The red ear represents simple inflammation of the tympanic membrane... Pain management is all that is needed not antibiotics.

94) B) When conjunctivitis and acute otitis media present together, the likely pathogens are beta lactamase resistant organisms, making amoxicillin/clavulanic acid the most appropriate treatment of those listed.

95) C) The history is most consistent with gonorrhea pharyngitis and a throat culture for gonorrhea would be the most appropriate step in establishing a correct diagnosis.

ER

96) D) Labial adhesions are rarely, if ever, related to sexual abuse; a crescentic hymen is a normal variation; and a normal genito-anal exam is frequently present in the face of sexual abuse and certainly does not rule out sexual abuse.

Tears that occur in the 3-9 O'clock/posterior position are more likely to be secondary to a tear. This is because a common variant of a normal hymen lacks tissue above the 3-9 O'clock/posterior position. Therefore this would not necessarily be diagnostic for sexual abuse. The exception to this would be previous documentation that hymenal tissue was present above the 3-9 O'clock/posterior position previously.

97)   C)   This is a classic history of a **breath-holding spell**. If it had been anything more significant they would have had to include more specific red flags in the clinical vignette. A history of cyanosis is typical of breath holding spells, not seizures. Cyanotic breath-holding spells are often preceded by something that makes the child frustrated or angry. However, this may not always be a part of the presenting history. In addition to the cyanotic spells, there are "pallid" breath-holding spells which are often preceded by a precipitating even. A diversion might be the child passing out right after being given an intramuscular injection. The injection would not be the cause but the emotional upset would be.

Some children who are prone to breath-holding spells have responded to treatment with Iron 6mg/kg/day even with no clinical evidence of anemia. In fact, those who are not anemic have been known to respond better to treatment.

98)   E)   Most cases of sexual abuse are perpetuated by someone well known to the family if not a family member themselves. Physical evidence of abuse is not always present and its absence does not rule out sexual abuse. Transmission of sexually transmitted diseases is not uncommon.

99)   D)   Anteromedial tibia, 2 cm distal to the tibial tuberosity is the correct location. It is important to go 2 cm below the tuberosity to avoid the growth plate. The other choices are incorrect, especially mid sternum (ouch!).

A chicken bone might be one of the correct answers since this is where the intraosseous line is placed during PALS training.

100) 1) (E)
2) (D)
3) (B)
4) (A)

There are specific clinical presentations which will be described which should make the diagnosis obvious on the exam,

Acute intermittent porphyria will be presented as paroxysmal abdominal pain along with headaches, dizziness, and syncope.

Ureteropelvic junction obstruction will be described as *recurrent episodes of periumbilical and midepigastric crams with episodic vomiting.*

Dysmenorrhea will be described as cramping midline abdominal pain.

Psychogenic pain due consistent with a conversion disorder will be described along with a psychiatric history in the patient and/or the family such as a labile patient and/or a depressed parent.

101) D) In most *hypertensive emergencies,* the drugs of choice are intravenous labetalol, nitroprusside, or sublingual nifedipine. **Patients with reactive airway disease are not able to tolerate a beta-blocking agent,** and beta-blockers are not the best treatment for hypertensive emergencies.

102) E) The first step in answering this question is to put the vital signs into descriptive adjectives. For example, this teenager is bradycardic and experiencing respiratory depression. This patient has the classic triad of opiate or narcotic ingestion **coma, pinpoint pupils, and respiratory depression.**

103) B) The technetium bone scan would be the most appropriate study to note any occult fractures missed by standard x-ray study.

104) B) Mannitol works via osmotic diuresis to reduce blood volume, and therefore works by reducing "brain water volume" overall.

105) D) Acute respiratory distress syndrome (ARDS) is a serious complication of "near drowning" in children. It is an uncommon complication, but is quite common on the boards.

The signs of ARDS may not be noted initially. During this "latent period", you may note mild respiratory distress, i.e., tachypnea, and perhaps an increased oxygen requirement. This is why "near drowning victims" who have required CPR in the field need to be admitted and observed even if they are clinically stable when they present to the ER.

On the initial physical exam you may note clear breath sounds or scattered rales. This is often followed by a typical deterioration as described in the vignette.

106) E) Anytime you are presented with the combination of bloody diarrhea and seizure you should think *"Shigella"*. You can remember this by changing to "Shakella" to help remember that seizures can result in a child with *Shigella.*

107) A) With the exception of the child with purpuric lesions noted on the lower extremities, the other scenarios are consistent with non-accidental injury. Purpuric lesions on the lower extremity would be consistent with Schönlein-Henoch purpura, which is often mistaken for child abuse.

Any history of multiple fractures in the absence of an underlying condition such as osteogenic imperfecta would suggest abuse. The other injuries could not be explained as an accidental occurrence.

108) C) In any acute trauma scenario, follow the ABC rule, with "A" being Airway assessment and management. This is another case where reading the question is critical to see what they are asking. The key word here is "Initial". Had they asked, what is the "initial radiological" study to perform; it would have been computed tomography or C-spine series.

109) C) Bruises can from accidental rather than intentional abuse can be identified by location of the bruise for example the shins in toddlers. Minor injuries can indeed represent a pattern of abuse.

The age of bruise cannot always be determined by the color alone. Other factors including depth of injury, location and the skin color of the child also influence the color of the bruise.

Cultural healing practices such as "coining" have been well described and should be factored in when examining a child for possible abuse.

Burn marks in a splash pattern would be more typical of accidental injury rather than intentional immersion which would more typically present with a sock and glove pattern.

110) A) With a supracondylar fracture, there is a 1% chance of vascular compromise and a 7% to 10% chance of a radial or median nerve injury. However, these injuries do not involve the growth plate. They typically occur in a child who falls on an outstretched arm. They can present with pain in the forearm due to vascular compromise of the brachial artery, and attempts to extend the fingers results in pain.

These signs are more reliable than the presence or absence of a radial pulse. Therefore, *a supracondylar fracture is not ruled out with the presence of a radial pulse.* **Do not eliminate supracondylar fracture just because they note the presence of a radial pulse on physical exam.** Prompt orthopedic intervention is needed when this injury is suspected.

111) A) When injury to the abdomen is suspected (as is the case in the clinical scenario presented), an abdominal CT with contrast would be the most appropriate NEXT step. Serial hematocrits might be a good idea, but not the next step.

112) E) Surprisingly in a household with 50 or more episodes of domestic violence taking place nearly 100% of children in these households will be physically abused.

113) C) The team trainer plays an important role in making sure the correct protocol for returning to full activity is followed. Clearly it wouldn't be the coach whose priorities might not coincide with the player. It would also help if the trainer is larger and more intimidating than the coach.

Mouthguard use in addition to preventing dental injury also provides some protection against concussions as well.

Most concussive episodes in young athletes are *not* reported. Regarding the management of concussions, the presence and resolution of symptoms are much more important factors than the assigned grade of concussion.

114) D) In any serious injury the ABCs takes priority. Therefore "assess airway" would be the most important initial step when assessing a fallen player with a potential cervical spine injury.

If the airway is compromised the facemask should be removed, while keeping the neck stabilized. **The helmet should never be removed in the field.**

In addition, you might want to note that the sport with the highest risk for cervical spine injury is football.

115) D) Rest, ice, compression, and elevation (RICE) are the most helpful 48 hours after the ankle injury. The most common cause of ankle injury is premature return not improper shoes or poor training. Fracture of the **5th** metatarsal is commonly seen with inversion injuries. This should be obvious if you simply inverted your foot while answering the question.

Heat should not be applied initially after an injury. Cold packs, once again, should be applied for 48 hours following the injury as a part of (RICE)

116) C) Fentanyl has no anxiolytic properties and therefore must be used with an anxiolytic agent such as midazolam. Therefore it is used for procedures which are painful and would have a limited or no role in a procedure which is merely distressing and not physically painful.

Fentanyl has a shorter half-life than morphine and therefore, morphine would be more appropriate for a procedure that will be painful afterward.

Fentanyl definitely does play a role in conscious sedation in children. Why else would you be expected to know about it?

Fentanyl, if titrated too quickly or given in doses greater than 5 mcg/kg, can result in chest wall stiffness.

117) D) As tempting as it might be, reassuring comments such as "I'm sorry we have to do this" have been shown to increase not decrease anxiety in children about to undergo painful procedures.

Cartoons, breathing exercises, video games and music all are helpful distractors to reducing pain and anxiety during procedures.

If you chose A, B, C or E, "I am sorry to have to tell you that your chose the wrong answer", which is no more reassuring than getting a letter from the Board of Pediatrics that begins "We regret to inform you that … blah, blah … you may take the exam again next year."

118) A) 90% of allergic reactions to food in children are due to one of the following 6 allergens, milk, eggs, soy, fish, wheat and peanuts.

Serving a tofu, cheese, salmon, peanut omelette served on whole wheat bread would require inclusion of epi-pens with the table setting.

119) C) The most likely explanation for this clinical presentation would be Mallory Weiss tears. Bleeding due to a Mallory Weiss tear typically follows forceful vomiting and/or coughing in the absence of abdominal pain. When abdominal pain does occur it is usually due to the musculoskeletal impact of the forceful vomiting / coughing episodes.

120) A) Cyclic vomiting is by definition stereotypic recurrent episodes of nausea and vomiting with no identifiable organic cause. There are several features required to establish the diagnosis including, 3 or more episodes of recurrent vomiting and intervals of normal health between episodes. There also must be a lack of lab or radiographic evidence to support an alternative diagnosis.

However amitriptyline and propranolol are effective *prophylactic* treatment. Antiemetic agents must be used during acute episodes.

Fluids & Lytes

121) A) Some of you might have remembered something about a ratio of 3:1. However that will only get you as far as narrowing it down choices A and E.

The correct answer is 3:1 glucose: sodium. Glucose: sodium ratio *greater than* 3:1 results in an increased risk for osmotic diarrhea. Another important piece of information is the glucose content, which should be 2-2.5% with a sodium concentration of 60-90 mEq/L.

122) D) With ***acute*** hyponatremia resulting in seizures, the goal is to *rapidly raise the serum sodium concentration by 3-6 mEq/L over a few minutes*. Free water is inappropriate. Remember it is 3% Saline NOT 0.3%. They have been known to play a number and decimal point shell game to trick you.

123) C) Hypernatremia results in the intracellular generation of idiogenic osmoles in brain tissue. This is to maintain homeostasis between intracellular and extracellular fluids. With correction it takes several hours for this to reverse and if the serum sodium concentration were to be changed too rapidly, fluid would rush in and cause cerebral edema and, subsequently, seizure.

124) E) This is a seizure secondary to hyponatremic dehydration. The treatment of choice is a hypertonic solution, which would be 3% sodium chloride. The target is to raise the sodium level high enough to stop the seizure; serum sodium of 125 mEq/L would be the goal.

Phenytoin could possibly stop the seizure, but it would not be the answer they are looking for in this scenario since it would not address the underlying cause of the seizure.

125) A) Given the sugar, salt, and water the child was given, one could surmise that he has hypernatremic dehydration.

As a result of the increased plasma osmolality, water shifts out of brain cells and into the blood. However, to prevent intracellular dehydration, these cells produce idiogenic osmoles such as taurine, myo-inositol, glutamine, and glycerophosphorylcholine.

These substances can remain in the cells during rehydration correction. If correction occurs too rapidly there will be excess movement of water into the CNS cells. Subsequently there may be development of cerebral edema, the most plausible explanation for the seizure.

126) E) This is a typical history and description of hypernatremic dehydration; therefore, the serum sodium concentration of 165 mEq/L is the best answer.

127) B) *Hyperkalemia* is an associated electrolyte abnormality seen with HUS. The toxin impairs absorption of sodium by intestinal cells in villi leading to hyponatremia. In addition the toxin causes cell death, resulting in the movement of potassium from intracellular to extracellular space leading to hyperkalemia.

Endothelial cell injury is an important component of HUS, leading to platelet aggregation and consumptive thrombocytopenia.

Metabolic acidosis and hyperphosphatemia are also seen in HUS.

128) E) Metabolic owing to poor tissue oxygenation would be the only logical answer since the carbon dioxide is not in a range to result in acidosis secondary to CO_2 retention. Decreased pulmonary function at the small airway level results in poor oxygenation leading to lactic acid accumulation secondary to anaerobic respiration and resulting in **increased acidosis at the tissue level.** There is nothing to suggest a renal or cardiac cause Excessive carbon dioxide loss would result in alkalosis, not acidosis as suggested by the pH of 7.25.

129) D) In the face of hypernatremia idiogenic osmoles are produced by CNS tissue to maintain fluid volume. If hypernatremia is corrected too quickly for the idiogenic osmoles to fade away, it could result in cerebral edema.

CNS is the only tissue where idiogenic osmoles are produced. In most, but not all, cases the testes are not a part of the CNS.

130) A) Hypernatremia is always synonymous with hyperosmolality. However hyponatremia does not always imply hypoosmolality as would be the case in acute or chronic renal failure.

Ethanol and methanol rapidly diffuse across cell membranes, so they do contribute to total osmolality, they do not lead to the movement of fluid across cell membranes.

When BUN is chronically elevated intracellular and extracellular concentrations are equivalent and urea does not contribute to effective osmolality.

131) B) Hypertension is frequently seen in Cushing syndrome. Edema is rarely seen. One would also expect so see increased body weight and serum sodium within normal range.

132) D) Pneumonia, asthma, salicylate toxicity, and pulmonary edema can all result in respiratory alkalosis.

Barbiturate toxicity would result in respiratory *acidosis.*

133) D) Spinal cord injury, myasthenia crisis, Guillain-Barré syndrome and botulism are associated with acute neuromuscular disease and can cause acute respiratory acidosis.

Nicotine toxicity is more likely to cause respiratory *alkalosis*.

134) D) Hyperventilation and dyspnea are seen in severe acidemia. Arteriole dilation and insulin resistance are also seen in the face of severe acidemia.

Cardiac contractility is decreased not enhanced in severe acidemia.

135) D) Diarrhea, pancreatic fistula, hypoaldosteronism, and renal tubular acidosis are all causes of metabolic acidosis with a *normal anion gap*.

Ethylene glycol toxicity is associated with a metabolic acidosis with an *elevated anion gap*.

Genetics

136) B) Down syndrome secondary to standard trisomy and Down syndrome due to translocation are phenotypically indistinguishable. While women older than 35 are at greater risk for having a child with Down syndrome, women in their 20s have more children with Down syndrome, simply because women in this age group have more babies. Had the question asked which age group has the higher "percentage" of babies with Down syndrome, clearly it would be women older than 35.

If the mother is carrying a translocation, the risk of recurrence is higher than if the father was the carrier. If neither parent is a carrier, the risk of recurrence is only 1%.

137) E) You would need to first know that glucose G6PD deficiency is an X-linked recessive disorder. Therefore, females are carriers since they have 2 chromosomes.

However, those with complete androgen insensitivity syndrome (CAIS)[8] are phenotypically female but genetically male. Therefore, they can indeed inherit X-linked recessive disorders like G6PD deficiency.

Complete androgen insensitivity syndrome could be the best explanation for a *phenotypic female having* a disorder which is inherited in an x-linked recessive pattern.

Of course this would not be the only way a female can get an X-linked recessive disorder. It could also occur if a female received both X-linked recessive genes from each parent.

However complete androgen insensitivity syndrome would be the *best* explanation.

138) B) You may not know or care to know about the details of the sequence or even what the q27 is referring to. The reference to the X chromosome should make the question simpler than it appears. Keep in mind that on the general pediatric board exam they would not expect you to know esoteric references to something discussed in the darkest caverns of genetics meetings under candlelight.

All you need to know here is that you have a "male" patient diagnosed with mental retardation and there is something "going on" with the X chromosome. That would tell you that the patient has fragile X syndrome. You could then rephrase the question to **"Which of the following are associated with fragile X syndrome?"** and then the answer is clearly macroorchidism, which is not a "big deal".

139) A) Since it is an "X-linked" recessive disorder, a male child who is unaffected does not have the genetic material. That is to say, there are no male carriers, and boys either have the disease or they don't and they are not carriers.

It is easy to get mislead and distracted into thinking the question is "additional children" in the existing family and not about future grandchildren. If you did not read the question carefully you would have found yourself "swimming with the red herrings".

---

[8] This was previously known as testicular feminization.

140) A) Children with Cri-du –Chat syndrome present with epicanthal folds, cardiac defects, psychomotor retardation and *micro*cephaly . They do not present with *macro*cephaly.

141) D) Russel Silver syndrome is associated with cardiac defects, abnormalities in the 5th finger, triangle face with normal head circumference. However wide spaced teeth are not part of the syndrome.

142) C) The description is classic characteristics of Cornelia de Lange Syndrome.

143) E) With macroglossia, hemihypertrophy, cardiomegaly, and hepatomegaly are all consistent with a diagnosis of Beckwith-Wiedemann syndrome.

144) C) The broad thumb and great toe should be enough information to make the diagnosis. Throw in the beaked nose and cardiac abnormalities and answering this one correctly should be a piece of cake.

145) C) The karyotype most associated with Klinefelter syndrome is XXY not XYY and it is the leading cause of male infertility. Males with Klinefelter syndrome are at increased risk for developing breast cancer. While children with Klinefelter have normal intellectual ability it is considered to be *slightly decreased* compared to the rest of the population.

Testosterone replacement is part of the treatment. Other features of Klinefelter syndrome include tall stature with long arms and leg, mildly delayed motor and language development, and a "calm demeanor". They may be described as being shy and sedentary.

146) B) Valproic acid can result in neural tube defects, short palpebral fissures, short nose, and straight contour to the upper vermillion border, cardiac defects, and mental retardation

ACE inhibitors can impact renal development negatively. Warfarin can lead to marked nasal hypoplasia and stippling of the epiphyses. Carbamazepine use, especially during the first trimester, increases the risk for neural tube defects, small short nose and small fingernails.

Heparin is considered to be safe during pregnancy.

An important fact to keep in mind is that fetal alcohol syndrome has physical features that overlap with exposure to anticonvulsants however fetal alcohol syndrome also results in babies being SGA and microcephalic.

147) D) The features described are a result of malformation as a result of mechanical forces which one would expect with oligohydramnios.

None of the other choices could explain the described features...

148) D) TEF is considered to be a "multifactorial trait". Since this cannot be traced to a single gene the specific genetic pattern cannot be identified. However there is an increased chance of conceiving a 2nd child with the defect than in the general population. The risk for conceiving another child with the same defect is 4%.

Single malformations due to a multifactorial inheritance pattern are the most common type of major anomaly seen. Other examples include pyloric stenosis, Hirschsprung disease, cleft lip with cleft palate, cleft lip and spina bifida.

149) E) Exposure to ACE inhibitors would best explain the findings of patent ductus arteriosis and fetal anuria.

150) D) The combination of thyroid disturbance and atrial septal defect would be consistent with fetal exposure to lithium. In addition infants exposed to lithium are at risk for Ebstein anomaly.

GI

151) D) A low fat diet can contribute to non-specific diarrhea and therefore one of the steps in managing this condition is to increase fat in the diet. Therefore 2% milk could be a contributing factor. Switching to whole milk would be one way to manage help resolve the problem. Excessive bile acids can contribute and juices that have fructose concentrations *in excess* of glucose can also contribute to the condition.

152) B) Cholestyramine and bismuth subsalicylate would be indicated if green stools were a part of the clinical picture; these would serve to bind fecal bile acids, a contributing factor in this form of diarrhea. Grape juice and orange juice contain fructose and glucose in a 1:1 ratio, which makes for better absorption of both. In addition, they contain no sorbitol, a major contributing factor to chronic non-specific diarrhea. On the other hand, pear and apple juice have high fructose to glucose ratios AND sorbitol, a double whammy. Fat intake and dietary fiber should both be **increased**, not decreased.

153) C) A family history of irritable bowel syndrome, peptic ulcer disease, as well as **previous appendectomy and migraines are more common in children with RAP**.

An onset of age *younger than 4* would require a more aggressive workup for a structural abnormality. Prognosis is worse among females than males. School absenteeism is a common problem but encouraging full participation in all activities including school is the best treatment; therefore, a private tutor would not be the best option.

RAP is a "functional disorder" because the exact pathogenesis and etiology of the pain is not clear. However, there are diagnostic criteria that must be met, and therefore it is not technically a "diagnosis of exclusion". The pain is usually episodic, a pattern in relation to meals and/or bowel habits is rare, and on physical exam the location of pain is usually vague.

154) 1) B
    2) C
    3) D
    4) A

An elevated ESR would correspond to the presence of chronic inflammation. Pernicious anemia could be seen on a routine CBC as macrocytic anemia.

Abnormalities of carbohydrate absorption could be assessed by measuring stool pH.

Disorders caused by disruption of the integrity of the intestinal lymphatic system could be diagnosed with a D-xylose absorption study.

155) C) The combination of bilious vomiting on all initial feedings along with a non-distended abdomen would suggest an upper GI obstruction distal to the pylorus. The double bubble sign would correspond with duodenal atresia and is the most likely diagnostic finding.

156) B) Irritable bowel syndrome is often precipitated by stress, resulting in recurrent diarrhea as well as crampy abdominal pain. Short stature is not part of the picture. While the presence of mucus in the stool is typical, hematochezia is not.

157) C) Indeed, here one has to read the question carefully. One would expect to find a sausage-like mass on the *right upper quadrant,* not the left lower quadrant. Bloody stools may not present until the first 12 hours, and this child became symptomatic 6 hours ago. Bilious vomiting can develop in patients with intussusception, and it is the most common cause of intestinal obstruction in children of age 3 months to 6 years.

Treatment of choice is air contrast enema, which is both diagnostic and therapeutic. Recurrence can occur 10% of the time, which means it does not in 90% of cases.

158) A) Ariboflavinosis is the deficiency of riboflavin. **Riboflavin's other name is vitamin B$_2$.** Ariboflavinosis is associated with **photophobia, blurred vision, burning** and **itching of the eyes, corneal vascularization, poor growth,** and _**cheilosis,**_ which are cracks and sores on the outside of the lips. Xerophthalmia is excessive dryness of the cornea and conjunctiva, caused by a deficiency of vitamin A.

159) C) The explanation should simply state that recurrent diarrhea in this clinical setting is most suggestive of _Giardia lamblia._

160) E) One would expect a patient to be low in albumin if they either:

Cannot produce it: End-stage liver disease

Cannot take it in: Kwashiorkor or other forms of malnutrition. _Intestinal lymphangiectasia_ resulting in obstruction of intestinal vessels would also impact absorption

Lose it in the urine: Nephrotic syndrome

Lose it in the stool: Inflammatory bowel disease, protein losing enteropathies, celiac disease, or GI infectious diseases

However, hepatitis A would not result in end-stage liver disease nor would it result in hypoalbuminemia.

161) B) This would be consistent with a history of _Gilbert's disease_, which is an _autosomal dominant_ disorder seen primarily in male. It is a benign disorder whose primary manifestation is a mild elevation of unconjugated bilirubin during times of high stress, such as physical training. One way to remember this is to think of a male named "Bert" with "gills" that gather in yellow dye, making him look yellow. This will help you remember that it affects males, the name Gilbert, and that it results in yellow color.

162) A) A *younger age of onset* represents a higher risk potential for developing hemolytic uremic syndrome after infection with enterohemorrhagic *E. coli.* Antimotility meds[9] should not be used since they can increase risk for hemolytic uremic syndrome in the face (no pun intended) of diarrhea.

Antibiotics can result in the increased release of the "vero toxin" when the *E. coli* cells are lysed.[10] Indeed, some studies have even suggested that toxin *production* could be increased. **Therefore, treatment with antibiotics would not be the correct choice when asked how to manage hemolytic uremic syndrome.**

Elevated WBC and prolonged disease are both poor prognostic signs as well.

163) C) The key here is the recent use of amoxicillin. They could have mentioned the recent use of any antibiotic, which can lead to *pseudomembranous colitis.* This is where writing notes in the margins comes in handy. Remember, the disease can occur weeks after antibiotics have been discontinued. A toxin produced by *Clostridium difficile* is responsible.

Treatment involves stopping any antibiotics the patient is currently taking and starting oral metronidazole. *This is now the drug of choice to reduce the incidence of vancomycin-resistant Enterococci.*

Vancomycin would be used if there were *no response to metronidazole.* In addition, no treatment is needed initially if the patient is currently on antibiotics and the symptoms stop after the antibiotics are discontinued.

164) D) Alpha 1 antitrypsin deficiency is the most common genetic cause of both chronic and acute liver disease in children. It is also the most common genetically caused disorder requiring liver transplantation in children. It can present as neonatal hepatitis syndrome in children.

Mild elevation of transaminase values can be seen in toddlers.

165) D) Since this infant is asymptomatic other than intermittent emesis and is growing well all that is necessary is reassurance

It is always more appropriate to have the infant sleep in the supine position to reduce the risk of SIDS. Thickening formula or medications would not be appropriate in this setting

---

9 Also known in some parts as the chemical plug.
10 The toxin largely responsible for the syndrome.

166) E) Non-bilious vomiting is typically seen in rotavirus infection. Rotavirus is typically seen during the winter months and often can include respiratory symptoms.

If you are presented with a child with bloody diarrhea, a diagnosis of rotavirus gastroenteritis will lead you down the primrose path of an incorrect answer.

167) B) The most recently licensed vaccine against rotavirus is a live vaccine which should be administered at 2, 4, and 6 months of age. The 1st dose should not be given later than 6-12 weeks of age and the 3rd dose no later than 32 weeks of age.

The risk for intussusception for the most recently licensed vaccine was similar for vaccine and placebo cases.

GU

168) D) Ocular chlamydia infection and chlamydia pneumonia in the newborn period can be obtained during the birth process.

However, a chlamydia vaginal infection in a pre-adolescent girl is almost always due to sexual abuse.

Malodorous vaginal discharge is frequently due to a foreign body (for example, toilet paper);

Anterior hymenal tears may not necessarily be due to sexual abuse. Tissue missing above the 3-9 O'clock position or the anterior position is a common normal variant. Therefore what may be described as a hymenal tear may actually be missing tissue within the context of this being a normal variant. Posterior hymenal tear is more likely to be due to sexual abuse.

Anal and vaginal penetration rarely occurs "accidentally". Straddle injuries are usually very painful often resulting in a crush injury of the penis or clitoris. *A straddle injury is usually brought to immediate medical attention and the child has full recollection.*

Condylomata acuminata can be obtained during the birth process and may not reflect sexual abuse; and likewise bacterial vaginosis can be seen following sexual abuse but it is nonspecific because it can be the result of rubbing in the genital area.

169) D) The symptoms are consistent with **torsion of the appendix testes.** It typically presents in a child between 2-11 years of age. The inflammation typically resolves within 3-10 days, and **surgical intervention is typically not indicated.**

170) D) If one simply followed the "least invasive procedure is usually correct" rule, it would have been simple enough to select the correct answer. Since the physical examination is normal an MRI study is unnecessary.

Since there is no mention of nocturnal enuresis, DDAVP therapy on a PRN basis is not necessary. DDAVP is reserved for occasional use when staying dry overnight is absolutely necessary for social reasons, for example a sleep over at a friend's house.

Since this child was toilet trained and assumed to be fully continent for the past year, the most likely diagnosis and first thing to be ruled out would be a urinary tract infection; therefore, a urinalysis would be the most appropriate next step.

171) D) The only explanation for bilateral, painless scrotal swelling which transilluminates, in an infant would be hydrocele.

172) E) A foreign body is commonly responsible for vaginal bleeding in preadolescent females particularly if it is described as malodorous.

In this patient, the foul-smelling discharge makes a vaginal foreign body, such as toilet paper, the most likely explanation. This is a frequently tested point on the exam.

173) C) In up to 1/3 of cases Henoch Schönlein purpura can present with acute pain, erythema and swelling of the scrotum especially in boys younger than 7.

Henpecked shoreline purpura is beyond the scope of this discussion indeed.

Heme Onc

174) C) Clotting factor 8 is not vitamin K dependent. Memorize the vitamin K dependent factors, 2, 7, 9 and 10; they always ask this. There is nothing more to it than that.

175) C) Pre-B cell type is the most common subtype and the one with the best prognosis. Rapid initial response to treatment corresponds to a good prognosis. Choices A and B are associated with a poor prognosis.

176) A) With a child with **unilateral disease** the chances are roughly **5%** that another child will have the disease; with **bilateral disease** the chances jump to **50%.**

177) E) An exchange transfusion *can* reduce the incidence of stroke, which occurs in 6% of patients with sickle cell disease. CVA's are due to both small and large vessel injury and focal strokes can result in subtle neuropsychological deficits. However, MRI, not CT, provides the most accurate diagnostic assessment by providing better image resolution than CT. MRI also is more sensitive in identifying subtle parenchymal changes common just after a stroke has occurred.

178) D) Neutrophils are the first line of defense of skin and mucous membranes against the rest of the world while fungal and other infections may occur. The best answer is choice D skin and GI flora. Treatment in the face of fever and other toxic signs in a neutropenic patient should be directed toward these organisms.

Likewise if they were to ask what the most common way neutropenia presents is, the correct answer is oral mucosal ulcerations and gingivitis.

179) D) If you are given no other information then viral syndrome is the most likely cause of neutropenia for a patient in your practice.

180) 1) (C)
   2) (B)
   3) (A)
   4) (D)

In **iron deficiency anemia,** the **TIBC** is high. Think of iron binding capacity as "trucks" to transport iron where it is needed. When there isn't a lot of iron around, as is the case with iron deficiency anemia, there are plenty of truck waiting around and the iron binding capacity is high. Serum iron stores or serum ferritin is low in iron deficiency anemia.

However, with **anemia of chronic illness,** there isn't a lot of iron around. The trucks don't have any gas and they remain in the garage, so the iron binding capacity is low. Since the reserves were there before the illness, **serum ferritin** is high in anemia of chronic illness.

It is easy to distinguish Beta thalassemia from iron deficiency anemia. The RDW will be high in iron deficiency and low in beta thalassemia

Serum **FEP** (free erythrocyte protoporphyrin) is elevated in both **lead poisoning** and **iron deficiency**. However, TIBC is elevated in iron deficiency and decreased in lead poisoning.

181) 1) (A)
   2) (B)
   3) (A)
   4) (D)
   5) (B)
   6) (D)

G6PD deficiency is an X-linked recessive disorder that is associated with **Heinz bodies.**

Howell-Jolly bodies are associated with sickle cell disease.

While hereditary spherocytosis is an example of a hemolytic anemia, it can also be associated with an **aplastic crisis** in association with a **parvoviral infection.**

182) 1) (C)
2) (D)
3) (D)
4) (A)
5) (B)
6) (D)

Thrombocytopenia is seen in both Wiskott Aldrich Syndrome (WAS) and Idiopathic thrombocytopenic purpura (ITP).

Eczema is only seen in Wiskott Aldrich syndrome.

Only ITP can be seen following a recent viral illness.

Increased PTT, abnormal platelet *function* and increased risk for malignancies are not seen in ITP or WAS.

183) 1) (A)
2) (B)
3) (A)
4) (B)
5) (D)

Joint pain is typically associated with JRA.

However, bone **pain**, lymphadenopathy and hepatosplenomegaly are more typical of leukemia. The increased incidence of leukemia with exposure to microwave towers has never been proven, so this is another popularly held myth that might steer you wrong on the Boards.

184) D) Whenever you are presented with a child who was "delivered at home," you have to assume that Vitamin K IM was not given. In addition the infant is 12 days old and has not been examined by a physician yet. You must consider hemorrhagic disease of the newborn up there on the differential, or sepsis if they present you with a scenario consistent with it.

In this case, the most likely diagnosis is *hemorrhagic disease of the newborn.*

A moderate decrease of the vitamin K-dependent factors[11] normally occurs in all newborn infants by 48 to 72 hours after birth. This transient deficiency of vitamin K-dependent factors probably is due largely to the absence of bacterial intestinal flora normally responsible for synthesis of vitamin K. In addition, **breast milk is a poor source of vitamin K,** and hemorrhagic complications have appeared more commonly in breast-fed than in formula-fed infants.

Warning: This is one of the few cases where formula would have an "advantage" over breast milk. This classic form of hemorrhagic disease of the newborn is responsive to vitamin K therapy.

Henoch Schönlein purpura is unlikely in this age group and with this presentation.

185) C) **While Fanconi's anemia is a congenital disorder, the pancytopenia typically isn't noted until the child is older than 8.** It is inherited in an autosomal recessive pattern. In addition to affecting blood cells, the disease affects the skeletal system[12] and results in abnormal skin pigmentation and kidney abnormalities.

Fanconi's anemia is also associated with chromosomal fragility.

186) D) The classic presentation of neuroblastoma in childhood would be an abdominal mass, perhaps coupled with raccoon eyes (periorbital ecchymoses). However, the tumor can also appear in the mediastinum. Neuroblastomas are tumors of the sympathetic chain. When it appears in this area of the body, the tumor can cause compression of the recurrent laryngeal nerve and the cervical sympathetic chain, resulting in Horner's syndrome.

---

[11] Factors II, VII, IX, and X. memorize these; it is frequently tested on the exam.
[12] Hypoplastic thumbs and aplasia of the radius.

187) B) *Iron deficiency anemia* is a microcytic anemia; therefore, the MCV will be reduced. **Both the serum ferritin levels and the serum iron levels are reduced.**[13]

In iron deficiency anemia, the serum iron binding capacity is actually increased, not reduced. The treatment of course is with iron supplementation.

The following table should help you keep this straight.

Anemia	Ferritin	TIBC
Chronic Illness	Normal or High	High
Iron Deficiency	Low	High

188) B) Given that 22 light years is a distance and not a period of time, this is easily ruled out. Cyclic neutropenia is characterized by regularly recurring episodes of neutropenia, typically lasting 3-6 days. In between these neutropenic episodes is a period of about 3 weeks.

This is similar to the timing and duration of menstrual cycles, which should help you remember this otherwise difficult fact.

These patients can present with oral ulcers and lesions, as well as adenopathy. They may also present with chronic periodontitis.

Consider this diagnosis carefully when presented with a patient presenting with unusual pathogens such as *Clostridium perfringens.*

---

[13] Note that in the anemia of chronic illness the serum iron level is reduced but the serum ferritin level is increased.

189) E)   Burr[14] and Helmet cells, as well as schistocytes, are all associated with hemolytic uremic syndrome.

Aaron Burr was the 3rd vice president of the U.S. who is better known for challenging Alexander Hamilton to a duel and mortally wounding him. Alexander Hamilton however has been immortalized on the $10 bill.

You can remember that schistocytes are associated with hemolytic uremic syndrome by picturing Aaron burr "shisting" a sword into Alexander Hamilton's kidney. Picture Burr wearing a "helmet" to remember that helmet cells are also associated with hemolytic uremic syndrome.

The **Coombs test** *can be* positive when hemolytic uremic syndrome is caused by pneumococcus, but **it is not positive with "typical" hemolytic uremic syndrome.** Again, reading the question for key words is important.

190) C)   This is a normocytic anemia making iron deficiency anemia unlikely. Folate deficiency is a macrocytic anemia and therefore also unlikely.

The high reticulocyte count findings and the fact that this child is black places sickle cell anemia high on the differential.

Therefore hemoglobin electrophoresis would certainly be the most logical next step in establishing the correct diagnosis.

191) E)   Severe anemia, hypersplenism, growth retardation, and chronic fatigue could all be indications for a transfusion. Extramedullary hematopoiesis however could be an indication for a splenectomy.

192) E)   Elevated serum unconjugated bilirubin elevated lactic dehydrogenase, and low serum haptoglobin levels all support a diagnosis of hereditary spherocytosis. However these are non specific and would be seen in any hemolytic anemia. Spherocytes can be seen in any case of immune mediated hemolysis including ABO incompatibility. In this case the direct Coombs would be positive in hereditary spherocytosis.

---

[14] Okay so it isn't really Aaron Burr cells. We took poetic license for the sake of humor.

193) B) A cholecystectomy is done in patients with hereditary spherocytosis if gallstones are present *only if they are painful, otherwise symptomatic or are causing bile duct obstruction.*

Gallbladder ultrasound is indicated every few years *after age 5.* This is recommended even if the patient is asymptomatic

A cholecystectomy is done at the time of splenectomy *only if gallstones are found preoperatively on ultrasound.* However it wouldn't be done routinely at the time of splenectomy.

194) E) Females and younger age at diagnosis are both factors which increase the risk of cardiotoxicity in children on anthracycline. Cardiotoxicity can occur with relatively lower doses.

However screening is done every 1-5 years depending on *cumulative dose.*

195) B) Secondary malignancies are especially common in survivors of Hodgkin's lymphoma. They are at particular risk for developing AML, Non Hodgkin's lymphoma and breast cancer.

196) E) The history and presentation is consistent with a diagnosis of G6PD deficiency with the antibiotic serving as the oxidative stress.

197) A) Wilms tumor typically presents as a painless abdominal mass often in an asymptomatic patient. Typically it is noted by the parent while dressing or bathing the child

198) B) A child with painless abdominal pain along with systemic symptoms especially the periorbital ecchymoses leads us to neuroblastoma as the most likely diagnosis.

199) E) There are no absolute hemoglobin or hematocrit levels that trigger consideration for a blood transfusion. Clinical conditions drive the decision. However Estimated traumatic blood loss or surgical blood loss of 15% would be considered triggers for a blood transfusion in the absence of physiological compensation.

ID

200) C) **The 3 C's of measles are cough, coryza, and conjunctivitis** Patients are contagious from 2 days before becoming symptomatic until 4 days after the onset of the rash.

While hand washing is a good idea with any infectious disease, measles is spread by droplets of respiratory secretions so **isolation** is the key to preventing the spread of disease not hand washing.

Encephalitis is not a common complication; it is a rare complication, affecting 1:1000 cases, and is insidious in onset not acute in onset. Subacute sclerosing panencephalitis occurs up to a decade later.

Measles specific IgM levels would be helpful if obtained **2 weeks later**, not at presentation. In addition, it is important to always consider measles when you see the word *coryza* in the history.

201) E) Pregnant women should not receive this live vaccine. However, children who are HIV positive and asymptomatic with high CD4 value should receive the vaccine because the benefits outweigh the risks. HIV patients with low CD4 values should not receive the MMR vaccine because vaccine related pneumonia have been reported.

A symptomatic HIV patient should receive IG prophylaxis regardless of immunizations status

Any individual born before 1957 would likely be immune the vaccine would be helpful only if given within **3-days (72 hour) of exposure**. A child who is younger than 12 months might not develop a strong enough immune response and should therefore receive immunoglobulin. So watch for an age younger than 12 months, and an exposure longer than 3 days earlier, in the wording of the question. Such children would not benefit from vaccination. However a 12 month old who is unimmunized would benefit from vaccination.

202) A) Rubella is actually a very mild disease. **In fact, routine vaccination is really to prevent disease in pregnant women and is the only vaccine given to provide protection for someone other than the child on the receiving end of the needle.** It is so mild that in the pre vaccine era, the disease was often inapparent.

The period of communicability begins 2 days before the appearance of the rash and lasts another 7 days. Infants with congenital rubella are considered contagious through body secretions up to *1* year after birth. Therefore F "could be true" so it is not the correct choice and besides I threw in the Oktoberfest line to remind you that rubella is also known as German measles, but Rubella is the term they will toss around on the Boards.

203) A) Children with pertussis are most contagious during the catarrhal stage. Unfortunately this is when suspicion is lowest because the symptoms are quite vague: cough, low-grade fever, and excessive tear production.

This will be described as cough, coryza, and lacrimation. Most cases of pertussis in the United States occur among unimmunized preschoolers or adolescents and adults whose immunity is waning, not infants who have not been fully immunized yet. *Maternal antibodies do not cross the placenta.*

204) E) Remember the RIP mnemonic. Confirmed cases of tuberculosis consists of treatment with isoniazid, rifampin and pyrazinamide.

205) E) Administration with BCG can result in a false positive result not a false negative result. All of the other choices can result in a false negative.

206) D) Bacillary angiomatosis and bacillary peliosis are seen in *immunocompromised* patients with CSD. Here is a case where you might read the question too carefully and misread the word immunocompetent.

It is not necessary to remove cats from the home to prevent future disease. The best prevention for CSD is the elimination of fleas.

207) C) Serum antibody for *Bartonella henselae* would not be any more important in the initial management than downloading the Mp3 for Cat Scratch Fever and both are incorrect. On the exam they will often present a cat bite or cat scratch and lay down the trap leading you to erroneously choose answers related to cat scratch fever.

The rapid onset of symptoms makes cat scratch disease unlikely. The incubation period for cat scratch disease is usually 3 to 30 days, with lymphadenopathy occurring in 1 to 4 weeks? In this case, the scratch occurred too recently (yesterday).

The patient is afebrile, and therefore a blood culture would not be a priority. However, a culture of the wound would be appropriate in this patient to identify the cause of the localized infection. The CBC with differential would provide evidence of the severity of infection. The most likely diagnosis is a simple puncture wound infection.

Since the cat is well known to the family, rabies status is not that critical since it could be assumed that the cat is immunized. However, checking the immunization status and seeing whether the cat is a house cat or one that roams the streets would be important. But it would *not be the first thing in managing this case.*

208) C) The rapidity of onset and intensity of local pain, swelling, and erythema are characteristic of *Pasteurella multocida* infection. This organism is associated with up to 80% of cat bite infections and is found in the mouths of approximately 65% of cats. *P. multocida* would likely be resistant to penicillin, making it an inappropriate choice. First-generation cephalosporins have limited activity against this organism. Amoxicillin/clavulanic acid would be effective against *Pasteurella multocida.*

209) B) Herpes simplex virus grows readily in cell culture, and special transport media are available for specimens that cannot be inoculated immediately. Serologic tests generally are not helpful for the diagnosis of acute HSV infection.

210) B) With community acquired MRSA becoming more pervasive , the most appropriate initial treatment in this setting would be trimethoprim with sulfamethoxazole.

211) E) Despite the findings consistent with otitis media, a full sepsis workup including lumbar puncture is indicated. Therefore, PO amoxicillin would not be appropriate. In this age group you must provide coverage for group B *Strep, Pneumococcus, Meningococcus,* and *Listeria* monocytogenes. IV ampicillin for *Listeria* and gentamicin for the other bugs would provide appropriate initial coverage until a bacterial infection has been ruled out or an organism identified.

In addition ampicillin and gentamicin would have a synergistic effect against Listeria.

212) E) Whenever you see the combination of
· renal problems
· anemia,
· thrombocytopenia,

You should automatically think of hemolytic uremic syndrome (HUS). This often manifests with fragmented RBCs and a high BUN and creatinine.

Young children are at greatest risk when exposed to the etiological agent.[15] It occurs after exposure to contaminated food, typically undercooked meat, although it can be contracted from dairy products and vegetables as well. Antibiotics are **not** routinely indicated nor are agents that stop the diarrhea. These can both make the situation worse.

213) B) The clinical scenario presented, staccato cough, diffuse infiltrates, and increased eosinophilia in an afebrile infant of this age, is most likely *Chlamydia trachomatis.* PO erythromycin would be the most appropriate treatment.

214) B) Azithromycin would be indicated for all household contacts as well as other close contacts *regardless of immunization status.*

The indication is controlling the spread of infection.

---

[15] *E. Coli* 0157:H7 for those into such details.

215) C) It is important to receive proper treatment within 2 weeks of exposure to the index case, *not 3 weeks*.

Beyond 2 weeks after exposure, immune globulin is not indicated since it will probably not be effective. Serological testing of close contacts is not indicated since it is not cost-effective and may delay administration of immune globulin in those cases where it is indicated. Hepatitis A vaccine would be indicated prior to traveling to an area where one would be at risk for contracting hepatitis A, *not post-exposure*.

Hepatitis A would not be indicated for *all newborns* of mothers with Hepatitis A. This is actually controversial and some suggest treating newborns *if* the mother is symptomatic 2 weeks before and 1 week after delivery.

216) B) Aminoglycosides such as gentamicin can result in blockade at the neuromuscular junction. Therefore, gentamicin and other aminoglycosides should be avoided in patients with underlying neuromuscular disorders.

217) E) You would need to know two facts here. One, the *P falciparum* species is chloroquine resistant. This poses a challenge when managing children, and it was a good punt by the internist.[16] Mefloquine might be the treatment of choice but it is contraindicated in children weighing less than 11kg.

However, this case is further complicated by the baseline seizure disorder. In such cases, mefloquine is contraindicated.

Doxycycline would be another option for prophylaxis but it wasn't one of the listed choices.

Atovaquone-proguanil is approved for children weighing less than 11 kg and would be appropriate for P falciparum prophylaxis.

218) D) CMV, adenovirus, Human herpes virus (HHV)-6 and rubella can present with a clinical picture similar to EBV infectious mononucleosis.

Paramyxovirus, does not present with such a clinical picture.

In particular, CMV, a frequent flyer on the exam, can also include atypical lymphs on the CBC. Look for hints in the question that EBV is the incorrect answer and CMV is the correct choice.

---

[16] Not really a punt since it was appropriate.

219) D) Discarding the box when it is ? full is the rule of thumb.[17] When it comes to recapping needles, one hand is better than two because of the increased risk of missing and getting stuck.[18] When they work right,[19] retractable needles are the better option. Needles and sharps should never be passed to another person, and the sharp container should be accessible to health care staff but not patients, especially pediatric patients.

220) B) This is an example where reading the question is critical. The question asked for the most common "cutaneous" manifestation, while condylomata lata is *a* manifestation of secondary syphilis, not a "cutaneous" manifestation. Condylomata lata are gray-white wartlike lesions found on mucous membrane tissues.

221) A) Among the choices given, CMV is the only correct one. Somewhere in the recesses of your board preparing cluttered mind you say you recall that rubeola also can result in deafness. Well, if rubeola "rings a bell" it is because sensorineural deafness can occur with congenital ru*bella* infection. It is very easy to avoid confusion in the future if you picture the "bell" in rubella ringing loud enough to cause deafness and loud enough to get the correct answer on the exam. In other words, when you see rubella as one of the choices a "little bell" should go off in your head. Rubeola should not.

222) D) You may have remembered Fitz Hugh Curtis, but it is also important to remember that this is *perihepatitis* and not hepatitis. The combination of joint symptoms coupled with right upper quadrant pain should help you identify gonorrhea as the correct answer.

Fitz Hugh Curtis can also be a manifestation of chlamydia infection as well.

223) D) Whenever a "park cleanup" is involved, "bird droppings" should be considered a prime suspect in the etiology of the presenting symptoms. In such cases you are down to two choices, histoplasmosis and coccidioidomycosis. With coccidioidomycosis, they will often describe and/or emphasize a headache.

---

[17] Pun intended.

[18] Just think of the paperwork alone.

[19] When is that?

224) B) An infant with lesions on the hands and feet along with hepatosplenomegaly would most likely have congenital syphilis. The decreased movement of the extremities is known as "pseudoparalysis" and the anemia is a "hemolytic" anemia.

225) C) If you are presented with a school aged child with clinical signs of pneumonia, especially with fever and malaise with a chest x-ray demonstrating bilateral diffuse infiltrates, you should consider a diagnosis of mycoplasma pneumonia.

The best treatment for mycoplasma would be azithromycin.

226) D) Full disclosure of the HIV positive status of to the day care center is *not* mandatory. Instead universal precautions must be in place precisely for this reason. Eczema and occasional epistaxis are not reasons for a child who is HIV positive to not attend the center.

Since stool and urine are not considered routes to transmit the HIV virus, children who are HIV positive and not toilet trained need not be separated from other children.

However HIV positive children with uncovered exudative skin lesions need to be separated from other children as well as HIV positive students who are excessively aggressive including those who bite and scratch.

227) C) You would need to cover for beta lactamase producing organisms including non typeable H. flu and M. catarrhalis. Using even higher dose amoxicillin won't help since they already noted that high dose amoxicillin was used. Azithromycin will not be effective against beta lactamase producing organisms.

Cipro and tetracycline would not be appropriate in a 7 year old and the argument stops there.

228) A) Clindamycin, Trimethoprim/sulfamethoxazole, linezolid and vancomycin are all appropriate choices for the initial treatment of methicillin resistant Staph aureus infections. Amoxicillin/clavulanic acid would not since these organisms are not sensitive to it.

Please note that the antibiotics listed would be appropriate for *initial* treatment only. There is increased resistance to these antibiotics and sensitivity must be established.

229) B) Rifampin is the mainstay prophylaxis for exposure to meningococcal sepsis. Any healthcare worker who examined the patient's throat or intubated the patient would be considered to be a close contact in need of prophylaxis. The appropriate dose for an adult would be 600 mg BID for 2 days. The maximum dose is 600 mg therefore 1200 mg q day for 4 days would be incorrect.

Ceftriaxone 250 mg IM would be okay but who would want a shot when one dose of ciprofloxacin can be given. It was important that the question stated that this is a male resident. Had it been a female resident the possibility of pregnancy would exist and ciprofloxacin would be inappropriate.

The meningococcal vaccine can be given as an adjunctive treatment in addition to antibiotics if it is due to a susceptible strain. Serotype A is a susceptible strain.

A, C, Y and W-135[20] are all susceptible strains.

230) C) The most common mode of transmission is via contaminated food. Mothers of affected infants are usually symptomatic with flulike symptoms a few days prior to delivery. However, there is a later onset form of listeriosis where the mothers are asymptomatic. However in early onset disease, which is the more common form mothers are usually asymptomatic.

Contrary to the species name monocytogenes, there is no monocytosis associated with listeriosis nor is there monocytopenia or leukopenia. However leukocytosis is an associated finding.

231) C) Listeria is always resistant to cephalosporins and therefore cefotaxime and ceftriaxone would be inappropriate. Ampicillin would of course be inappropriate in a penicillin allergic patient.

Chloramphenicol has a high failure rate and has side effects that would make it inappropriate. Trimethoprim –sulfamethoxazole is bacteriocidal and reaches good levels in the CSF.

---

[20] Why are they called, A, C , Y and W-135? Do you care? Just remember these are the susceptible strains!

232) E) Maternal IgM titers, positive amnionic viral cultures and positive polymerase chain reaction all will help establish congenital CMV infection which was already given to you in the question.

However this would not help predict the neurodevelopmental outcome.

Likewise, documented hearing deficit following maternal *recurrent* CMV infection would suggest that even the hearing loss won't be progressive. The outcome is generally better with recurrent CMV disease than with primary CMV disease.

233) E) In a routine case of CSD in an immunocompetent patient the appropriate treatment is nothing more than supportive care. Lymph node biopsy would be reserved for atypical cases and cases where diagnosis cannot be confirmed by any other means.

234) A) Incubation periods are *shorter* in children. Patients on chronic steroids, or who sustain bites closer to the CNS and/or multiple bites can expect a shorter incubation period. The mean incubation is 30-90 days

235) D) While one could argue that A "Beam me up Scotty I have one for Mr. Spock" is correct it would not be the best answer, although very logical. You would have to read the question and more importantly write down what each serum marker means in words.

For example:
HBsAb = Hepatitis B Surface antibody.
HBsAg = Hepatitis B Surface antigen
HBcAb total = Hepatitis B core antibody (total IgG and Ig M)
HBcAb IgM = Hepatitis B core antibody acute phase

This makes it much easier to interpret with Spock-like rational interpretation devoid of any emotion.

In this case the HBsAb is negative , therefore the patient is not immune. Therefore any choices referencing immunity is logically incorrect.

Therefore you are down to 2 choices chronic or acute infection. Since the HBcAb/ IgM is elevated you are dealing with an acute infection leaving you with the only logical choice, choice D, "Acute hepatitis B infection".

236) B) While one could argue that choice E is correct which spells out "Help, my eyes are so glazed over moths have been landing on my eyes without my noticing" would be correct it shouldn't if you just follow the moth to the light.

If you are asked a question regarding the "replication rate" or "infectivity" of hepatitis B, then you are dealing with the e antigen.

You are either dealing with: HBeAb (antibody) or HBeAg (antigen). Clearly a high rate of replication or infectivity would be associated with a high HBeAg (antigen) level.

So now that you see the light, hopefully the moths will follow suit and leave your eyes and head to the light themselves.

237) C) While one could argue that choice E is correct which spells out

"How the heck should I know" is the correct answer? However, you really should know as follows:

You can easily narrow your choices down to the 2 with HBsAb positive. If the HBcAb is negative then the patient would be immune due to vaccination. If the HBcAb is positive, the immunity would be result of recovery from acute infection which is choice C.

Now you should be asking "Howtheheckcanlgetthiswrong?" = "How the heck can I get this wrong"?

Metabolic

238) E) Patients with homocystinuria, sulfite oxidase deficiency, Fabry's disease and ornithine transcarbamylase deficiency all are at increased risk for cerebral vascular occlusion. Patients with tyrosinosis are not.

239)   A)   Hunter's syndrome is X-linked recessive. This is best remembered by envisioning hunters using X's at the end of their bows and arrows when they hunt. In addition most hunters are male and X-linked recessive disorders affect males.

240)   1)   C
2)   B
3)   B
4)   A
5)   D

Both Hurlers and Hunters syndromes present with course facies. Only Hurlers presents with corneal clouding after all you can't see if you are a hunter and is autosomal recessive.

Hunter's syndrome is X-linked recessive. Skeletal involvement and normal intelligence would describe Morquio syndrome which is not included in this question.

241)   E)   Phenylketonuria (PKU) is the most plausible explanation for the situation described in the question. In the real world it would be unusual for a patient to present at 6 months due to diligent screening required by law. However, this is the Boards, a world unto itself. It is recommended that the blood for screening be obtained after 48–72 hours of life and preferably after feeding proteins in order to reduce the possibility of false-negative results

242)   B)   Ornithine transcarbamoylase deficiency is a urea cycle defect and therefore would indeed be associated with elevated serum ammonia levels. Elevated serum ammonia levels are also seen in methylmalonic acidemia.

Reye's syndrome and other diseases associated with liver failure result in elevated serum ammonia levels.

Like Reye's syndrome, Leigh disease is also associated with encephalopathy; however, it is not associated with elevated serum ammonia levels.

243) E) The vignette describes **Lesch Nyhan syndrome**, which is categorized by self-mutilation. Because of the abnormal movements, it can be confused with athetoid cerebral palsy. However, the choices point to a specific metabolic disorder and the typical features of Lesch Nyhan are being described. Please note that uric acid levels are for diagnostic purposes only. Bringing the uric acid levels under control will *not* help control any of the neurological or behavioral manifestations of the disorder.

244) A) The combination of physical and lab findings makes for a diagnosis of Van Gierke disease which is glycogen storage disease type 1. (GSD 1)

GSD I is due to glucose 6-phophatase deficiency which impedes the breakdown of glycogen into glucose.

This results in the **accumulation of glucose -6-phosphate.** → **increased lactic acid**

Hepatomegaly results with failure to thrive.

Elevated uric acid levels, ketonuria hyperlipidemia also result. Clinically seizures are also a common presentation.

Treatment is the frequent feeding of carbohydrates such as corn starch.

245) E) Most infants identified in newborn screening with elevated phenylalanine (PA) levels won't have PKU. In some cases it might be due to delayed maturation of metabolizing enzymes. Others might have biopterin deficiency.

The bottom line is infants identified in PKU screening require additional workup before concluding that they have PKU.

246) D) The patient's newborn screening and anterior fontanelle make hypothyroid unlikely. There is nothing to suggest myasthenia gravis, mitochondrial disorder or glycogen storage disorder, making for a most likely diagnosis of botulism poisoning. The introduction of cereal was mentioned for a reason. Honey might have been part of the preparation.

247) D) The combination of hemolysis, liver disease with preceding neurological signs makes for a diagnosis of Wilson disease and thus a serum ceruloplasmin would be the most helpful test.

Musculoskeletal

248) D) While this is an X-linked disorder, the mother is not **always** an asymptomatic carrier. Since X-linked recessive disorder is one of the other choices it may seem like the two are contradictory. Following the rule to never choose a question with "always" in it, you will likely get this correct.

While mothers are usually the asymptomatic carrier, there is also a high spontaneous mutation rate. **In up to 1/3 of the cases the mother is *not* the carrier.**

249) C) Since this is a girl where less than 2 years of growth is expected and the angle is less than 25 degrees, only watchful observation is needed and a follow-up film in 6 months.

250) C) This is a classic description of dermatomyositis and the treatment is with steroids.

251) A) A Salter-Harris I injury is a disruption of the growth plate only. It is a diagnosis often made on clinical grounds since the fracture can be quite subtle. Therefore, it is very likely that the injury from several months earlier was a Salter-Harris I fracture that was not diagnosed and this is a re-injury.

Conversion disorder? I don't think so!

252) D) Each of the signs listed are common findings with TMJ dysfunction except for swelling of the TMJ. Consider that snapping your gum excessively can also lead to TMJ dysfunction.

Excessive discussion of board questions with colleagues after you have already taken the exam can also lead to TMJ dysfunction followed by conversion reaction.

253) B) SCFE is the slippage of the epiphysis of the proximal femur in relation to the metaphysis. For those who do not feel comfortable with orthopedic Latin, this is simply the slippage of the femoral head. It often appears as an ice cream scoop slipping off the cone on x-ray, especially on the Boards.

SCFE often presents as referred knee pain, especially on the exam. Estrogen increases the strength of the growth plate, and both testosterone and growth hormone weaken the plate.

Therefore, elevated estrogen levels would not be a contributing factor. SCFE occurs more frequently in males and African-Americans than in Caucasians.

254) E) **Osteogenic sarcoma** and **Ewing's sarcoma** are not benign tumors.

Osteoid osteoma, while common on the Boards, is not the most common benign tumor seen in children.

Osteochondromas are outgrowths of normal bone as well as cartilage and are the most common benign tumors in children. However, their location is abnormal. These are confirmed on x-ray and removed when symptomatic or when risk for malignant transformation is present. Malignant transformation should be suspected when continued growth occurs after skeletal maturity is reached or there is a new onset of pain.

Osgood Schlatter's disease is caused by micro-fractures of the tibial tuberosity and is not a bone tumor.

255) B) Children with **achondroplasia** have normal intelligence. It can be inherited in an autosomal dominant fashion, although most cases arise from a new mutation to normal parents. Therefore, genetic testing is not always performed or necessary. While virtually all infants and children with this disorder are born with large heads, only a fraction have true hydrocephalus.

Lumbar spinal stenosis can present later in life, and loss of bladder and bowel control may be a late complication.

256) E) Bilateral calve pain occurring exclusively at night in the absence of systemic symptoms or physical findings is classic for growing pains

257) C) Legg calve Perthes disease is a self limited disease resulting from avascular necrosis of the capital femoral epiphysis. It frequently occurs in boys between ages 4-10. Onset before the age of 6 carries a better prognosis due to the extended period of time for bone remodeling.

Girls tend to have a higher prevalence of bilateral disease. However bilateral disease is not associated with more severe disease or a worse prognosis.

MRI is more helpful than x-ray during the early stages of disease.

258) C) The classic history of slipped capital femoral epiphysis (SCFE) is a teenager, usually obese who presents with minor trauma, with symptoms out of proportion to the trauma.

Although involves the hip joint, pain is often refereed to the knee. They present with the leg externally rotated and slightly flexed. Passive internal rotation is difficult due to pain

259) E) Idiopathic scoliosis is due to multiple factors and does not follow any specific inheritance patterns.

260) D) The appropriate order of diagnostic testing for Duchenne muscular dystrophy is

Creatinine kinase levels → genetic analysis → muscle biopsy

Clearly muscle biopsy is the most invasive and is last. Creatinine kinase levels would be a first initial screen. Molecular genetic analysis has advanced in recent years. These have reduced the number of patients receiving muscle biopsy unnecessarily.

A muscle biopsy would not be useful if creatinine kinase levels and genetic analysis are normal.

261) A) Are you getting the picture? More often than not the correct answer will be multifactorial when this is among the choices. This is not a hard rule and of course if you know that another choice is the answer then pick that one.

However when in doubt pick multifactorial as the answer.

262) D) The conservative or non surgical intervention of choice to treat congenital talipes equinovarus is casting and splinting.

Neonatology

263) E) Developmental dysplasia of the hip is more common among Caucasian babies than African-American babies. It is more common among females and full-term babies, as well as those delivered by breech presentation.

264) D) Omphaloceles are indeed associated with several anomalies, including Beckwith-Wiedemann syndrome. Additional associated findings of Beckwith-Wiedemann syndrome include macroglossia, macrosomia, and hypoglycemia

Failure of the umbilical ring to contract is associated with herniation of the umbilical cord. Folate-deficient diets during pregnancy have been linked to spinal cord defects, not omphalocele.

Gastroschisis is a similar defect. However, with gastroschisis there is no membranous covering and the defect tends to be smaller and is not associated with Beckwith-Wiedemann syndrome. .

265) D) Erythema toxicum is a common lesion in newborns. Diffuse pustules with an erythematous base characterize it. It would be distinguished from a *Staph* infection by the presence of eosinophils when the contents of the pustules are examined under the microscope.

Dry peeling skin is common in newborns, especially those who are post term. *Miliaria crystallina* are vesicles that are a result of the accumulation of sweat just below the skin surface due to sweat gland obstruction. It resolves on its own.

The *yellow papules* on the hard palate are *Epstein's pearls,* and these too are a common finding in newborns. This resolves in weeks.

On the other hand, a midline skin tag on the spine can be benign, but it can also be a marker for more serious defect involving the spinal canal. Therefore, radiological studies such as an MRI are indicated.

266) C) It is most important to avoid cold stress with its metabolic consequences. This is particularly important with a premature baby. Choice D can be done later on, once the infant has been stabilized and you have ingested a couple of Almond Joy® bars to wake yourself up. This is consistent with assessing airway first, since setting up optimal conditions for evaluating the newborn would be the first step en route to evaluating the airway.

267) E) The most important factor in determining bonding of father and child is presence in the DR. It enhances closeness with the mother and also insures bonding with the baby in the initial hours after birth. Due to such modern equipment like DVD players, ,and HDTV in delivery rooms, fathers can now be present and see the opening kickoff or the opening schtickoff on the Dr. Phil show.

Age is one of the factors. However, adolescent males tend not to bond as well. An estimated 80% of fathers are present for their baby's delivery; 95% is too high a figure and would include the fathers who attend c-sections with their video cameras.[21]

268) B) The correct answer is B. Here is a case where, as noted in our main text, it is important to put numbers into words. In this case, since you already know the diagnosis, it makes sense to place the description "hypochloremic metabolic alkalosis" in the margin as a reminder of the corresponding lab findings seen with pyloric stenosis. You could then at least begin eliminating choices with low bicarb and a high chloride. This is a lot easier than reasoning it all out. There is plenty of time for that after you are board certified and can afford to be "certified bored".

269) D) Pyloric stenosis, with its progressive projectile vomiting and loss of HCl in emesis, results in *hypo*chloremic alkalosis; it occurs primarily in male *first-born* babies; and there is usually a history on the *maternal* side.

It is always best to correct any metabolic abnormalities preoperatively, especially the alkalosis in order to reduce the risk for post-op apnea. I have known few pediatricians who have palpated the fabled olive and some pediatric surgeons who palpated the olive *and* the pimento, mostly at the bottom of a martini glass when they are at home post call. .

---

[21] I always wonder whom they are going to show this to. Guests that won't leave?

270) E) Since the mother was treated for eclampsia, it is likely that she was treated with magnesium sulfate, resulting in hypermagnesemia in the newborn. Watch for the proper spelling: hyper-*manganesemia* would not be a factor.

After the use of $MgSO_4$ within 24 hours of delivery, one should watch the newborn for signs of magnesium toxicity, including neuromuscular and respiratory depression

The mechanism to explain this is as follows: acetylcholine in the motor nerve terminals acts on the myocardium by slowing the SA node impulse formation and prolonging conduction time but this is way too boring and really should be in a well hidden footnote at the bottom of the page.

271) E) This is the classic presentation of "congenital torticollis", and early diagnosis and passive stretching is all that is needed. Proper management should result in significant correction within a few months. Otherwise, referral to orthopedics is needed to "set things straight".

One might also look for reflux as a potential cause of torticollis. Sandifer syndrome refers to the association of seizure-like posturing or torticollis as well as the presence of GERD. Often there is no vomiting with this, but it is quite amenable to anti-reflux medication and other precautions like positioning and thickened feeds.

272) C) The ABG is consistent with metabolic alkalosis and their mentioning the child's being on furosemide (Lasix®) is your clue. The fact that the child has BPD is not critical to the question. The question could have simply asked you to make a diagnosis based on the ABG alone. Lasix® results in metabolic alkalosis by decreasing chloride in the urine and increasing bicarb urine loss.

273) E) This is a description of pseudotumor cerebri, and too much vitamin A can cause it.

274) A) In total anomalous pulmonary venous connection, the pulmonary veins do not go back to the left side of the heart as they should. This is the underlying problem. Findings on x-ray include diffuse granular pattern due to increased pulmonary vascular markings. You might see the snowman sign or figure 8, but rarely before 4 months of age. This is due to cardiomegaly.

In early infancy you could see mild cyanosis, and signs of failure (dyspnea, tachypnea, tachycardia, and hepatomegaly).

There is no evidence of RDS or Group B Strep pneumonia. Cardiomegaly would not be a part of the clinical picture seen in transient tachypnea.

275) D) The clinical picture is a relatively benign one and is consistent with a diagnosis of transient tachypnea of the newborn which is self limited and improves with supportive care within a few hours.

276) B) Approximately 10% of newborns require some form of resuscitation in the delivery room. This would include requiring tactile stimulation and oxygen and even some bag/mask ventilation.

A newborn can be expected to establish regular respirations by 1 minute after delivery.

277) E) Placing the baby on the mother to allow for breast feeding is important during the first hour when the baby is alert. Vitamin K, erythromycin, height and weight measurement can all wait for this which should be given top priority even if the staff is due for their break in an hour.

278) C) Early discharge is considered prior to 48 hours after a vaginal delivery. For a C/section 72 – 96 hours. This is despite any HMO humming sounds.

Early discharge is only okay if the infant is feeding well, stooled and voided and all screening tests are completed. Most newborns void within 12 hours.

In addition, early discharge is not okay if the mother is GBS positive.

279) D) The American Academy of Pediatrics recommends that all infants discharged prior to 72 hours be seen within 48 hours (2 days). This is assuming the absence of risk factors.

280) D) Breast feeding jaundice which might be described as *"breastfeeding associated jaundice"* is due to initial poor caloric intake until milk "comes in". The decreased caloric intake is a stimulated entero-hepatic circulation resulting in indirect hyperbilirubinemia.

281) C) There is nothing in the history to suggest ABO incompatibility. Breast feeding jaundice is seen in the first few post natal days and the clay colored stools would not explain human milk associated jaundice or Gilbert syndrome.

The only diagnosis to explain the clay colored stools (acholic) is cholestasis.

282) D) *Conjugated hyperbilirubinemia* is defined as conjugated bilirubin greater than 2.0 or greater than 20% of the total bilirubin. Even though they are used interchangeably direct hyperbilirubinemia and conjugated hyperbilirubinemia are not considered the same. [22]

Unconjugated hyperbilirubinemia is more common than unconjugated and Gilbert syndrome is associated with unconjugated hyperbilirubinemia.

Conjugated hyperbilirubinemia is not always associated with cholestasis. Rotor and Dubin Johnson syndromes are two examples that are not associated with cholestasis.

283) C) If you break this question down, they are really asking you "What would be the first thing to do in managing a tachypneic infant with small muscle mass?"

There is nothing in the history to suggest fetal exposure to drugs therefore a urine tox screen would not be indicated.

Given the low glucose reserves of small infants and the fact that hypoglycemia could result in tachypnea; the answer is to obtain serum glucose. Again, the least invasive is usually the correct answer. While equally as non-invasive, obtaining electrolytes would not have the same yield.

---

[22] I doubt you will have to know why but if you are a glutton for punishment here goes, direct bilirubin may include both the conjugated fraction and bilirubin bound to albumin (delta bilirubin) and therefore .... Zzzzz. I think you get the picture.

284) E) This is a typical presentation of a trachea-esophageal fistula (TE fistula), probably with a blind pouch esophagus connecting to the trachea. This is the most common variety of TE fistula, and it presents as choking episodes with feeding and the production of copious secretions. A feeding tube will appear coiled up in the blind pouch-ending esophagus on x-ray.

There is nothing in the history to suggest choanal atresia; therefore insertion of a catheter into both nares and/or a CT scan would not be indicated.

285) C) Fetal tachycardia, hypertrophic cardiomyopathy, and hyperinsulinemia are among the known side effects of terbutaline. However the result of fetal hyperinsulinemia is neonatal *hypo*glycemia not hyperglycemia

286) A) Fetal exposure to indomethacin increases risk for oligohydramnios, periventricular leukomalacia, and necrotizing enterocolitis (due to cerebral and splanchnic vasoconstriction). There is also a risk for *reversible* not *irreversible* renal failure.

287) C) Gastroesophageal reflux can present with chronic wheezing and in sever cases failure to thrive. Regurgitation typically occurs 30 minutes after a feeding and irritability during or after feedings is a common finding.

However, the latest studies show that there is no proven beneficial effect of head elevation in the supine position.

288) E) Rumination is the repeated and painless regurgitation of ingested food into the mouth. Usually it occurs soon after food is ingested. It is often seen in cases of neglect and there is a strong behavioral / psychological component.

Symptoms do not occur during sleep , do not respond to standard treatment for gastroesophageal reflux and symptoms must be present for 8 weeks or longer to establish a diagnosis.

Rumination is *not* associated with retching.

Neurology

289) A) Lisch nodules, neurofibromas and optic gliomas are associated with NF type 1. Additional findings include boney defects such as intramedullary fibrosis cortical thinning and sphenoid bone dysplasia.

Learning disabilities are associated with neurofibromatosis type 1.

However acoustic neuromas are associated with neurofibromatosis **type 2.**

290) C) This is a trick question, which is not uncommon on the Boards, and requires a careful look at the wording of the question. While it is safe to reassure parents that a child experiencing a febrile seizure stands little chance of developing epilepsy, the chances still double from roughly 1 % to 2 % so choice B is true.

Therefore while the risk is still low it does double from 1 to 2%. Fair? Not really but who said board exams are fair?

The risk of epilepsy is irrespective of the number of febrile seizures the child experiences. Therefore choice C is NOT true. Neuroimaging is rarely indicated and lytes, glucose and even calcium should be reserved for cases accompanied by diarrhea.

While an "LP" isn't routinely indicated, meningitis must be ruled out "clinically" and if there is clinical evidence of meningitis an LP *would be appropriate.*

291) E) This is a typical description of partial complex seizures. School aged children are typically affected, and the episodes can start out with "staring spells", which then generalize and lead to "automatisms" such as clicking sounds. Family history can be negative, and EEG's are frequently negative. Treatment is with anticonvulsants.

Rolandic seizures typically occur at night, which helps differentiate them from partial complex seizures.

Absence seizures do not occur with automatisms and do not typically result in a post ictal picture. In addition, there are typical EEG findings. Therefore, if there is a negative EEG in the question, you can usually cross out absence seizures from the choices presented.

292) D) There is no evidence of trauma so subdural and epidural hematomas are ruled out.

Cardiomegaly and failure to thrive suggest congestive heart failure.

This would make a **vein of Galen malformation**.

Consider this diagnosis when they describe an infant with hydrocephalus and congestive heart failure.

293) 1) (B)
2) (C)
3) (A)
4) (D)

Absence seizures are associated with a 3 per second spike and wave EEG pattern.

Infantile spasms are associated with a hypsarrhythmia pattern on EEG.

Complex partial seizures would be associated with a child presenting with lip smacking.

Rolandic seizures typically occur at night and this should be part of the clinical description on the boards.

This can be remembered by picturing a child with rolandic seizures **rolling out of bed at night.**

294) 1) (A)
2) (F)
3) (B)
4) (D)
5) (E)
6) (C)

Chorea can be described as smooth movements of the extremities.

Rhythmic movements of the head would be a tremor.

Twisting, assuming postures would be a **dystonia**.

Brief muscle jerking movements would be **myoclonus**.

Brief movements of the face and shoulder would be a **tic**.

Excessive ants-in-the-pants-like movements would be a classic description of **hyperactivity**.

295) E) The clinical presentation is most consistent with a cerebral hemorrhage due to an *arteriovenous malformations* resulting from a failure of normal capillary bed development between arteries and veins during embryogenesis. Arteriovenous malformations produce abnormal shunting of blood, causing an expansion of vessels and a space-occupying effect or rupture of a vein and intracerebral bleeding. Arteriovenous malformations are typically located in the cerebral hemisphere.

Rupture of arteriovenous malformations causes a severe headache, vomiting, and nuchal rigidity due to subarachnoid bleeding, progressive hemiparesis, and a focal or generalized seizure.

296a) A) Myasthenia gravis typically presents with bulbar[23] and systemic weakness.

Multiple sclerosis would not typically present in this age group and neither would "infantile" botulism. **Polio** is rare and they would have to give you a clue such as lack of immunization and/or recent travel to a place where polio is endemic. Guillain-Barré presents with ascending[24] paralysis typically following a viral illness.

296b) B) The presence of anti-acetylcholine antibodies causes the disease. A positive edrophonium chloride (Tensilon®) test and EMG findings are diagnostic.

296c) E) A cholinesterase-inhibiting drug (anticholinesterases) such as neostigmine or pyridostigmine is critical in managing the symptoms of this disorder.

297) B) This is a typical description of *infantile spasms,* known previously by the politically incorrect term "salaam movements". This "visual", however, remains a simple way to recognize the presentation of infantile spasms. Keep in mind that infantile spasms may also present with tuberous sclerosis, so watch out for a description of both in the same patient.

The hypsarrhythmic pattern on EEG[25] is also characteristic of infantile spasms and gives away the diagnosis.

---

[23] By bulbar we are not referring to light bulbs. We are referring to bulbar weakness of the muscles innervated by the cranial nerves, manifesting in decreased extraocular eye movements, diminished gag reflex, and laryngeal muscle weakness.

[24] Legs first, and then "ascending" up to the face.

[25] Not to worry, you won't be presented with the actual pattern; you will just need to recognize the word.

298) C) With depressed consciousness and continued deviation of both eyes, this would likely be due to persistent seizure activity and should be treated as such.

A New York State of mind would be deviation of both eyes to the right.

299) E) The keys in this description were his having "no prior injury" and the assumption that he will remain asymptomatic. This would be categorized as a Grade 3 concussion because of the loss of consciousness. The minimal period of being symptom free is 1 week; therefore, had he been symptomatic he could not return to play. A head CT is mandatory since there is a history of loss of consciousness. In this case the fact that a head CT was done is noted in the question.

300) E) The combination of a transient focal headache with contralateral weakness would be consistent with a diagnosis of familial hemiplegic migraine. This is supported by the family history of migraine headaches.

301) B) A tic disorder would be characterized by a motor **or** vocal tic but not both. Sniffing which cannot be suppressed would be considered to be a *vocal tic* as would chirping sounds or throat clearing.

Children with Tourette syndrome have *both* motor and vocal tics, not necessarily at the same time but they both must be present to establish the diagnosis. They must occur daily for one year with no tic free period longer than 3 months.

Since the boy is alert during these episodes this cannot be absence seizures. There is nothing to suggest attention deficit hyperactivity disorder.

Although the boy is sniffing there is nothing to suggest allergic rhinitis. The eye blinking would constitute a motor tic. Therefore the combination of a motor and vocal tic would suggest a diagnosis of Tourette syndrome.

302) C) Children with epilepsy may take a bath or swim provided there is an adult supervision. Driving is permitted provided the patient on medication and seizure free for 3-12 months.

Obtaining an EEG is not useful in weaning a patient off of medications. The presence or absence of seizure activity is more important.

Juvenile myoclonic epilepsy requires lifetime treatment usually with valproate.

303) D) Onset of seizure before age 1, low degree of fever at the onset of the seizure increase the chances of having febrile seizures in the future. However they do not increase the risk for developing epilepsy.

Males who have a febrile seizure are not more prone toward developing epilepsy.

However a family history of epilepsy places a child at increased risk. In addition a child experiencing a complex febrile seizure would be at increased risk for developing epilepsy. The following factors would constitute a complex febrile seizure:

· Duration longer than 15 minutes
· Recurrence within 24 hours
· Focal seizure

In addition the following factors would also increase the chance of developing epilepsy in a child having a febrile seizure:

· Presence of neurological or developmental abnormality
· Febrile seizure on 3 or more occasions
· Fever for less than 1 hour before the seizure

Nutrition

304)   E)   Breast-feeding should continue through the first 6 months **and beyond** if possible. This is a trick choice because the AAP suggests *exclusive* breast-feeding throughout the first 6 months. Therefore "breast-feeding through the first 6 months is adequate" is not really a true statement since additional breast feeding through the first year would be more appropriate.

The components of breast milk are **not** constant at all during the first year. The components change to coincide with the nutritional needs during the first year. Breast milk contains **IgA** not IgG. This is another instance where reading the question carefully is crucial. At casual glance it is very easy to confuse IgA with IgG.

Human milk does **not** contain T cells and alpha interferon; however, there is strong evidence that breast milk complements the infant's own immune system via immunomodulation.

305)   D)   Human breast milk will provide phylloquinone, fluoride , vitamin D, and vitamin B12 can be found in breast milk under *most* conditions, However of the choices listed , only ascorbic acid (vitamin C) can be found in adequate amounts under *all* conditions.

Phylloquinone is also known as **vitamin K.**[26] Initially infants, even exclusively breast-fed babies, are at risk for vitamin K deficiency. These infants are therefore not good at producing vitamin K dependent factors (remember 2, 7, 9, and 10).

Exclusively breast-fed infants are also at risk for being vitamin D deficient if the mother is not getting adequate vitamin D in her diet and/or the infant is not getting adequate sun exposure.

As for fluoride, **fluoride *IS* found in breast milk**, *if there are adequate amounts in the water supply.*

However, it is important to note that the AAP recommends fluoride supplementation for infants over 6 months who are exclusively breast fed and are not getting fluoridated water.

Therefore if the question pertained to an infant younger than 6 months of age, choice B, would not have been true, either.

For all you strict vegetarians out there, remember to take B12 supplements. Vegetarians are at risk for being **B12 deficient** and therefore will not be providing enough in their breast milk if they are not taking B12 supplements.

---

[26] Remember to commit these fancier names to memory; they will employ anything to get you into the wrong side of passing.

306) 1) (C)
2) (D)
3) (B)
4) (A)
5) (A)

If freedom's just another word for "nothing left to lose" then ergocalciferol is just another name for Vitamin D_2 and cholecalciferol is just another name for Vitamin D_3.

25, hydroxy vitamin D is hydroxylated in the liver.

1, 25 hydroxy vitamin D is activated calcitriol and hydroxylated in the kidney.

307) 1) (C)
2) (A)
3) (B)

Essential fatty acid deficiency can result in → scaly dermatitis, alopecia, thrombocytopenia

Zinc deficiency can result in → dry skin, poor wound healing, perioral rash

Vitamin E deficiency can result in → hemolytic anemia, peripheral edema, thrombocytopenia

308) B) In "developed" countries such as the United States where the endemic rate of HIV infection is low and commercially available formula is a safer alternative, breast-feeding would be contraindicated, as would the use of pooled breast milk.

However, in "developing countries" outside the US where HIV is more endemic, severe poverty more common, and commercially available formula not as readily available, the risks of "not breast-feeding" and the subsequent risks of inadequate malnutrition may outweigh the risks against contracting the HIV virus from breast milk. That would be a more complicated question.

However this question is specific regarding protocol <u>in the United States where safe alternatives to breast-feeding are available.</u>

309) B) Medium chain triglycerides (MCT) *are* present in human milk and *some* infant formula.

However medium chain triglycerides are *not present in cow's milk*. They do *not* require micelle formation with bile salts for adequate absorption; this makes MCTs a good source of rapidly available metabolic fuel.

310) A) Biotin deficiency results primarily in dermatitis, and more specifically seborrhea. You can picture a "rusty **tin**" to remember that **biotin** causes skin problems to lock this into memory.

311) B) Oxaluria, the excretion of excessive amounts of calcium oxalate, can result from excessive intake of ascorbic acid or vitamin C.

Ascorbic acid taken in excessive dosages can also lead to nephrocalcinosis.

312) D) You would need to know that **cobalamin** is the formal name for **vitamin B12**, which is commonly deficient in a vegetarian diet. This concept is frequently tested on the exam.

It can also be an issue with a **breast-feeding mother** who is on a vegetarian diet. Vitamin B12 deficiency often results in megaloblastic anemia.

313) C) The clinical description is of a child suffering from retinol or vitamin A deficiency. Bumping into objects at night would be consistent with night blindness nyctalopia. The silvery patches on the eye are known as bitot spots which is also consistent with Vitamin A deficiency.

To avoid permanent blindness retinol supplementation is crucial.

314) E) The best explanation for *all* of the clinical findings in this patient would be Cystic Fibrosis.

Cystic fibrosis would explain repeated bouts of bronchiolitis as well as the foul smelling diarrhea which would be due to malabsorption.

Malabsorption would lead absorption of fat soluble vitamins. These would include Vitamin D deficiency which would explain the low serum calcium and elevated alkaline phosphatase levels. Low Vitamin E would explain the hemolytic anemia. Low vitamin A levels would explain the conjunctiva injection which would be due to follicular conjunctivitis.

315) A) Given the history of a home delivery and no mention of the infant being given Vitamin K the most likely explanation for the clinical manifestations would be hemorrhagic disease of the newborn due to factors, 2, 7, 9 and 10 deficiency.

The most appropriate treatment would be 2 units Vitamin K.

316) C) Both preterm and full term infants require 100-120 Kcal/ Kg /day to grow. In preterm infants this may be more difficult to achieve on standard formula which is why they require preterm formula which has more calories per ml.

317) B) The most common electrolyte abnormality during the first week of refeeding in a malnourished patient with anorexia nervosa is **hypo**phosphatemia. It is not clear what mechanism is responsible for that, but now you at least know what the correct answer would be. if this pops up on the boards.

318) C) The most likely explanation for the patient's clinical presentation would be Galactose-1-phosphate uridyltransferase deficiency resulting in *galactosemia*. Infants with galactosemia are prone to gram negative sepsis such as E. coli. Hepatomegaly, elevated indirect bilirubin and positive reducing substances all go along with a diagnosis of galactosemia.

There is a risk for development of cataracts and they should be fed soy formula.

Pharmacology

319) 1) (B) Acetazolamide.
  2) (A) Furosemide.
  3) (D) Hydrochlorothiazide.
  4) (C) Spironolactone.

320) E) Trimethoprim/ sulfamethoxazole would be the first line treatment for each of the conditions listed except for exacerbation of chronic bronchitis for which it would be considered to be a 2nd or third line medication.

321) C) Valerian root is used to treat anxiety and insomnia. Caution should be used when taking sedatives or drinking alcohol.

322) C) St. John's Wort is used as an antidepressant and its mechanism of action is postulated to be serotonin reuptake inhibition.

323) 1) (C)
  2) (G)
  3) (A)
  4) (A)
  5) (D)
  6) (F)
  7) (E)

Cyclophosphamide can result in hemorrhagic cystitis, therefore patient on this agent must be well hydrated. Patients on bleomycin need to be monitored for pulmonary fibrosis.

Both anthracycline and doxorubicin can be cardiotoxic. Vincristine is neurotoxic and asparaginase can cause pancreatitis. Methotrexate is associated with oral ulcerations.

Preventive

324) D) Drowning deaths and injuries occur 4 times as often in boys. The surrounding fence is a critical component to preventing drowning, a concept frequently tested on the exam. Infant and toddler swimming lessons, while cute and enjoyable for parents, has not been proven to prevent drowning. Children in this age group lack the ability of learning to swim and/or understanding safety issues; if anything, it gives a false sense of security.

In fact the AAP has a policy statement that swimming lessons should not be started prior to 4 years.

325) D) The most common agent for causing burns in children is hot liquid. This can occur either by immersion or via a spill. Spills occur primarily in children younger than 4 years.

326) C) Each of the choices is an example of a common myth with the exception of choice C. Had choice C read "10 days" of steroids instead of 12 then this too would have been another example of a pediatric myth. One of my favorites is choice E, the one about going out with wet hair. If this were true then all Olympic swimmers starting with Mark Spitz in 1972 would have been dead after one week of training.

Another common myth not listed is the need to wait (fill in the blank) hours before swimming after eating. I grew up knowing parents who had a grid listing the time you needed to wait depending on what you ate. Some items, like a hot dog, required that you stay out of the water 3 weeks. If you ate a burger and fries you were out for the duration of the summer.

Ref: Debunking pediatric myths. *Contemporary Pediatrics.* March 2001.

327) B) A sibling who is older than 6, whose immunizations are up to date, and who has received the latest booster within 3 years would need no additional immunizations. However, prophylactic antibiotics are necessary for all household contacts and other close contacts such as those who attend daycare with the index case.

328) C) Each of the choices is a rare complication of the varicella vaccine except for temporal lobe seizures. In addition to the side effects listed, Guillain-Barré syndrome and Stevens-Johnson syndrome have been seen after administration of the varicella vaccine.

329) D) The varicella vaccine is contraindicated in all of these situations except HIV-positive children who are *asymptomatic* or *mildly symptomatic*.[27] At the present time there are protocols whereby children with ALL can receive the vaccine *if they are in remission.* Those not in remission cannot receive the vaccine.

330) C) Necrotizing fascitis is a rare but life-threatening complication of *chickenpox infection*, not varicella vaccine. *Strep pyogenes* infection can be a complication of chickenpox, but not the vaccine. Acute cerebellar ataxia has been reported after and attributed to the vaccine itself and therefore would be the correct answer.

331) A) "Egg-Xactly."[28] Substituting egg whites (notice we did not say egg yolk) for fat is a good way to reduce fat/cholesterol in the diet.

Nonfat and low-fat milks are not recommended for use during the first 2 years of life because of lower caloric density compared with whole-fat products. Total cholesterol or HDL does *not* require fasting but calculation of LDL *does.*

Regarding puberty, there is an increase in cholesterol levels just before puberty and a decrease during the growth spurt.

---

[27] For those with a hand-held wireless slide rule this means a CD4 T lymphocyte count greater than 25%.
[28] As Vincent Price in the role of Mr. Egghead used to say, in the old Batman series.

---

332) A) The key to a correct answer here is memorizing the formula. In all likelihood, they will test you on either sensitivity OR specificity, but test on this concept they will. It is worth getting it straight so you can get one more question correct on the road to passing. The sensitivity of a test is the truly "positive results" over the total number with the disease, thus how "sensitive" a test is. Therefore it is:

[True positive test results] ÷ [Total with disease]

Just remember:

$$\frac{\text{True +}}{\text{Actual +}}$$

Total with disease would be all who have it, which are the *true positive* test results and the *false negatives.* In this case, the total number with the disease is 81 plus 37 = 118. The total positive test results are 81, and dividing this by 118 is roughly 0.68. Therefore, a very sensitive test (high number) will pick up a lot of patients with the disease and is therefore good for "screening". An example would be the rapid *Strep*, which is reliable when positive. Therefore, it makes good "sense" to use a sensitive test to "screen".

333) B) The sensitivity would be:

[True negative results] ÷ [Total without the disease (healthy)]

The total without the disease would be the true negatives plus the false positives (who are healthy). In this case, this would be 48 divided by (48 plus 5) 53 = 0.90.

This test is reliable to confirm the disease; for example *Strep* throat culture. Tests which have a high specificity, help confirm disease such as the throat culture for *Strep*.

334) E) This would be the positive predictive value, which is:

[True positives]   [Total positive test results]

Here you take the true positives and divide by the total number of positive test results (true positives plus false positives). In this case, it is 81 divided by (81 plus 5) 86 = 0.94. Positive predictive value is the chance of a person with a positive result actually having the disease.

As you might have guessed, the *negative predictive value,* which is not one of the choices here but could appear on the exam, would be:

[True negatives] + [Total negative results]

The *negative predictive value* is the number of true negatives divided by total negatives (true negatives and false negatives). In this case, this would be 48 divided by (48 plus 37) = 0.56.

Now that you have waded through these questions, you should have an approach with high specificity and a high positive predictive value.

Psychosocial

335) B) Emetine —the active ingredient in ipecac. Several keys in this question point toward Munchausen by proxy syndrome (MBPS). For one thing, she is ER-hopping in Central Connecticut despite the negative workup at what must be teaching hospitals in Manhattan.

A non-medical person using terms like "hypovolemia" and "capillary refill" is bizarre even for someone who has taken her kid in several times for a GI workup. One might argue that "maternal porcelain levels" would be the correct answer to diagnose a "crock". It is a tough one, but the questions do ask for the "best" answer to establish the diagnosis, not the most logical

336) 1) A
     2) D
     3) A
     4) B
     5) A
     6) B

Night terrors occur during the first third of the night and the child is mobile during the episode, making for the possibility of physical danger. There is usually no recollection of the episode. There is often a family history.

With Nightmares there are often vivid recollections of the nightmare. Neither one is associated with nocturnal enuresis. Abrasive commentator Tucker Carlson as president would be considered a nightmare.

337) E) While ADHD has no relation to diet, a well-balanced diet is appropriate advice for any child, regardless of diagnosis. There is no evidence that preservatives or any other food products including sugar causes ADHD

338) E) This is a description of "disfluency" and is a normal finding in a child of this age and something the child will likely outgrow naturally with time. This typically occurs at the beginning of the sentence, especially when the child is tired or being asked a question. No further workup, studies, or intervention would be warranted at this time.

Ankyloglossia is the formal word for "tongue-tied". Even if this were present on physical exam, it wouldn't warrant any further intervention.

339) C) Children with educable mental retardation[29] can expect to develop communication skills in the preschool years, although this is often delayed. They can be expected to read at a 3rd to 6th grade level and develop some vocational skills. Many remain self-supporting, marry, and go on to be successful parents.

Somebody with an IQ of 70 would be way overqualified to be an anchor on a political show on Sunday morning. Boredom would overwhelm them within a week.

---

[29] IQ in the range of 5 to 69.

340) D) The most common presentation for mental retardation is language delay. The more profound the retardation, the earlier this comes to the attention of parents, caregivers, and health care providers.[30]

341) D) Primitive reflexes are present at birth and through the first year of life, but are abnormal if they persist past that point. As the brain matures and an infant's development progresses, the primitive reflexes disappear as the infant gains fine voluntary motor skills. Persistence of primitive reflexes is seen in infants with cerebral palsy.

The *corneal reflex* is also known as the *blinking reflex*, where the eyes blink when touched or in the face of sudden bright lights. This reflext persists normally and is therefore not a primitive reflex.

In addition to the *step reflex* (touching the sole of the foot results in stepping motions; disappears at 1-2 months), other examples of primitive reflexes include:

Startle reflex – with drawing of the arms and legs in response to a loud noise

Moro response – elicited by partially lifting the upper body and letting go, resulting in the startled infant throwing its arms up

Parachute reflex – elicited by rotating the baby from supine to prone quickly, resulting in the infant putting its arms out

Tonic neck reflex – elicited with the infant laying supine and by turning the head to the side; the arm on that side extends out with the hand opened and the arm on the opposite side flexes with the fist clenched (Picture a *fencer* position and remember it well; this has been included in the photo section of the certification exam, and you need to know that it is a normal finding.)

Rooting reflex – when the infant's cheek is stroked it turns to that side

Grasp reflex – just as it says, the infant grasps an object placed in its hand and won't let go (disappears at 3 months)[31]

Primitive reflexes are *always* normal in males. In fact studies have shown that the number of primitive reflexes is directly proportional to testosterone levels.

---

[30] In many cases also known as physicians or PCPs (primary care providers).
[31] Normally reappears at law school graduation.

342) A) Correction for prematurity should be done until the age of 2 years. In this case, if one adjusts for the 4 months prematurity and makes the assessment based on that of an **11-month–old**, then the mother need only be reassured since the milestones achieved would be normal for an adjusted age of 11 months. It would, of course, not be normal for a 15-month-old.

343) E) Head banging and thumb sucking in an 18 month would be normal developmental variant seen in up to 20% of children between the ages of 6 months to 4 years especially boys.

344) C) **Rolandic epilepsy** is characterized by seizures that occur at night. However, minor rolandic seizures are characterized by tonic clonic movements, often affecting one side of the face. A rolandic seizure typically begins at the corner of the mouth, and spreads to the rest of the face. Sometimes these seizures generalize to that entire side of the body. Clearly this is not occurring in the vignette.

Night terrors typically occur in boys between the ages of 5 and 11.[32] Night terrors typically occur during the first third of sleep during the *non-REM cycle.* Usually the child cannot be aroused and has no recollection of the event. Autonomic arousal manifested by tachycardia and tachypnea is typical.

345) D) There is often a lot of resistance on the part of parents to the diagnosis of ADD, and for good reason. There is a lot of misinformation out there and resistance for parents to accept and in some cases clinicians to make the diagnosis. On the other hand, the diagnosis is sometimes made flippantly, and stimulant medications are prescribed without employing the behavioral strategies needed to round out appropriate management.

Sometimes behavioral modification is employed without stimulant medication, often with poor results.

The **best approach** is to ease the parents into the diagnosis, reminding them that one can be successful.[33] A stepwise approach is best, with medication being discussed last, not first. Approximately 40% of children with ADHD will have an associated learning disorder, which may explain why the child in this case "doesn't like reading." This too must be addressed.

In fact AAP clinical guidelines require full neuropsychological testing to evaluate for other comorbidities.

---

[32] Thus it is always worth noting the gender of the patient.

[33] Adults with ADD tend to gravitate to fields like this father did because of the high level of stimulation and need for sustained attention.

346) C) The key to this answer is the fact that the child has remained on the 25% of the growth curve for 6 months and has not "fallen off the curve". Other than reassurance, no other steps would be necessary since the assumption would be that the child is getting adequate nutrition. Yes there is a tendency for reassurance to be the correct answer with questions on psychosocial issues.

347) E) Here, one would have to assume that the academic performance up until now has been fine, especially since they note that this deterioration was "recent". There is no evidence presented for focal brain abscess; hydronephrosis should not lead to uremia; and there is no evidence of a temporal lobe seizure or ADHD. Therefore, hearing loss secondary to recent aminoglycoside use would be the most logical choice.

Risk factors for aminoglycoside ototoxicity include: **therapy lasting more than seven days**, elevated serum levels, prior exposure to aminoglycosides, noise exposure, or high daily dose.

Therefore of the choices listed only hearing loss secondary to ototoxicity makes sense.

348) B) Sitting is usually achieved by 7 months, pincer grasp by 4 months, transferring objects by 6 months, smiling by 6 weeks, crawling by 7 months, and supporting weight and taking steps with assistance by 9 months.

These are all developmental milestones of an infant that has reached 9 months of age, but not that of a 12 month old. Therefore, the correct answer is choice B, 9 months of age.

349) E) This is a classic presentation of ADHD, a chronic condition that is frequently diagnosed around the first grade when greater demands are made. This child is exhibiting signs of hyperactivity[34] on physical exam. Difficulty completing homework assignments is an important feature of ADHD reflecting difficulty with organization skills.

Patients can often mask the signs during an initial evaluation. This is often not deliberate since the "novelty" of the situation is "stimulating enough" to keep the child focused during the evaluation.

Therefore, you cannot rule out ADHD in a child that sits still for the initial evaluation. In addition, on history the clinical signs must be present in at least two venues, typically at home and at school.

---

[34] Difficulty sitting still and talking excessively.

350) B) Clearly the mother is overextended and could use some assistance in handling her multiple responsibilities. Social work consultation would be most effective in developing strategies and tapping into resources that might reduce her stress level.

351) C) Children with special needs are at increased risk for physical abuse and neglect both at home and in educational and child care settings.

The divorce rate is *higher* than in families without a child with a special needs need.

Family members are at an increased risk for depression

352) C) Crying for up to 3 hours a day in a 6 week old would not suggest any specific organic cause.

However the crying which starts suddenly, is persistent and lasts for an hour or more is consistent with a diagnosis of infantile colic.

353) E) *Less than* 50% of parents enforce TV viewing limits for their children.

Around 50% of children 8 years and older have video games in their room and 70% have TV's in their rooms.

The TV is on during meals in around 65% of homes.

The AAP does recommend that children younger than 2 years of age not watch *any* TV

354) C) Studies have shown the strongest support for SSRIs such as fluoxetine when pharmacological treatment is necessary for the treatment of separation anxiety disorder in children.

Pulmonary

355) D) Bronchiectasis is a *permanent* dilation of bronchi or bronchioles in a particular segment of lung, resulting in recurrent infections involving the same lung segment. Symptoms often increase when the patient is lying down.

356) A) The best explanation would be persistent hypoventilation following hyaline membrane disease in this former premature baby. Therefore, measuring oxygen saturation during sleep would be the most appropriate next step.

357a) E)

The history, physical exam, and x-ray findings make pneumonia secondary to tuberculosis the most likely diagnosis compared to the other choices. Typical tuberculosis characteristics include fever, weight loss, fatigue, coughing, lymphadenopathy; crackles on lung exam Lab findings would include monocytosis. Chest x-ray should exhibit perihilar infiltrates.

357b) C)

Placement of a PPD would be the least invasive and most efficient method to confirm a diagnosis of tuberculosis.

358) B) Once again, a good rule of thumb is that whenever something is in quotes the diagnosis should be taken with a grain of salt. In this case, the infant is probably not having "choking episodes" and the pediatrician probably reassured the mother.

This is most likely nasal congestion, commonly seen in infants, and nothing more than reassurance is necessary. Therefore no need to wake him up and you can let the doctor continue his "sleep study".

359) D) Whenever the word "pneumonia" is in quotes this is a hint that it is being defined by the parent and is not the actual diagnosis, which is probably benign, post-tussive, and emissive. Recurrent "pneumonia" with wheezing is most likely reactive airway disease. Recurrent otitis media in and of itself would not suggest an immunological disorder. However, more than one hospitalization in a child this young for "febrile pneumonia" would suggest an immunological disorder, perhaps B agammaglobulinemia. Because of the hospitalizations you could assume that this was a pneumonia confirmed with lab, clinical, and radiological findings.

360) A) Definitive diagnosis of choanal atresia is by CT scan. The inability to pass an NG tube is only suggestive of the diagnosis.

Choanal atresia is a component of CHARGE association, which stands for coloboma, heart disease, choanal atresia, retardation, and genital and ear anomalies.

Infants are obligate nose breathers until the age of 5 months, and obstruction of both nares can be life threatening.. Therefore, an oropharyngeal airway can help facilitate mouth breathing.

361) C) A diagnosis of exercise-induced asthma is supported by an FEV_1 decrease of at least 15%. When reading the question make sure they are describing a 15% decrease in **FEV_1**

362) B) The clinical vignette described is of **moderate persistent asthma** manifested by periods of wellness interrupted by daytime and nighttime symptoms. Consultation with a pulmonologist would not be necessary and is rarely the correct answer on the exam.

The use of steroids via a nebulizer twice daily, and albuterol via a nebulizer on a PRN basis would be appropriate. **Chronic use of albuterol would not be indicated**. Instructions on the use of a peak flow meter to assess subclinical asthma would be appropriate.

In addition, *rhinitis and/or sinusitis often accompany asthma*, and treatment of these conditions can reduce the severity of asthma. Therefore, management of nasal congestion with intranasal steroids would be an important adjunct to the management of chronic asthma.

363) C) Inhaled corticosteroids used prophylactically help reduced asthma flare-ups by several mechanisms including the following:

Induce production of beta 2 receptor enhancing action of beta 2 agonists such as albuterol

Decrease the number mast cells in cells lining airway

50% of patients well controlled on inhaled steroids *still* experience exercise induced asthma

With conventional metered dose in inhaler, up to 80-90% of the inhaled dose is deposited in the oropharynx

Leukocyte protease inhibitor synthesis is **increased.**

364) A) Remember that "diagnosed by parents" in quotes often means it is a red herring. The history is consistent with recurrent reactive airway disease.

What the mother describes as "pneumonia" isn't necessarily pneumonia. Recurrent pneumonia described by the parents is often reactive airway disease.

The history is not consistent with a diagnosis of cystic fibrosis, absence of secretory component of IgA, or foreign body aspiration.

365) A) Pulmonary function testing will confirm that it is the peak expiratory flow rate or the forced expiratory volume in one second (FEV_1) that is decreased with asthma.

The testing is done immediately before exercise, immediately after exercise, and 5 and 10 minutes later.

366) A) Levalbuterol has not been proven to be superior to racemic albuterol as a first line bronchodilator in routine asthma exacerbations. Viral infections are implicated much more commonly as triggers than bacterial infections.

Regarding patients having a supply of systemic steroids at home, there are situations where this would be appropriate. Patients who have a history of repeated severe exacerbations can have a supply at home. In such cases starting treatment early has benefits provided it is done in coordination with the doctor.

Chest physical therapy and mucolytics have no role in the routine management of asthma exacerbations.

367) C) Mild intermittent asthma is

General symptoms less than 2 times a week

Night symptoms less than 2 times a month

In addition children whose asthma is only triggered by viral infections are considered to have mild intermittent asthma.

This is the only group for whom bronchodilators alone is appropriate treatment for acute exacerbations. There is no daily maintenance treatment.

368) E) Medium dose inhaled steroid plus a long acting bronchodilator

Medium dose inhaled steroid alone

Medium dose inhaled steroid and leukotriene modifier

Medium dose inhaled steroid and theophylline

Are all treatment options for moderate persistent asthma?

Inhaled cromolyn sodium would not be an appropriate treatment option for moderate persistent asthma.

369) D) Inflammation is the underlying abnormality present in patients who have even mild asthma.

Inhaled cromolyn prevents both the early and late airway response to *allergy triggered* asthma and inhaled steroids help inhibit the late but not the late bronchospastic response

Severe early bronchospasm responds promptly to short acting bronchodilators

Mast cell activation is responsible for the *immediate* bronchospastic response to allergen exposure.

370) D) The most likely cause of malaise, low grade fever, headache, dry cough and bilateral patchy infiltrates on x-ray would be mycoplasma pneumonia.

Renal

371) D) Post –strep glomerulonephritis, membranoproliferative glomerulonephritis, systemic lupus nephritis all are associated with low serum complement levels.

However rapidly progressive glomerulonephritis is not associated with low serum complement levels.

372) A) Medullary cystic kidney disease has a **gradual onset**, not an acute onset. Anemia, growth failure, polyuria, and polydipsia are common findings. It is a disease that involves pathology of the renal tubules, and progression to end-stage renal failure is inevitable.

373) D) There is nothing in the history to suggest any specific cause other than essential hypertension in this patient. Essential hypertension often runs in families, which is the reason the father's and the uncle's histories are mentioned.

By the way if they had not noted that the blood pressure was elevated on 3 separate occasions it is not hypertension by definition.

374) B) Prune belly syndrome more commonly affects males, and cryptorchidism is one of the associated findings that can be seen. While the urethral and vaginal structures can be involved in females, **ovarian dysplasia is not seen in prune belly syndrome**. Renal dysplasia and pulmonary hypoplasia are also typically seen.

375) D) This question is another example where writing down the meaning of the lab values in words is critical. In addition, when presented with the components of the anion gap, you need to calculate and note whether it is elevated.

Here the Bicarb is low and you are therefore dealing with a **metabolic acidosis**. If there were a respiratory component, you would have been provided with blood gas values. The sodium, potassium, and chloride are normal. The anion gap would be (136-114-10) = 12. The anion gap is within the normal range.

A normal anion gap rules out organic acids as the cause of the metabolic acidosis. There is no indication of genetic short stature since they do not mention the parents' heights, and they wouldn't give all these lab values if that were the diagnosis. Polycystic renal disease does not result in metabolic acidosis at all, so this choice is eliminated.

You are now down to proximal and distal renal tubular acidosis. Often, but not always, if you have these two diagnoses among the choices, it will likely come down to one of them. This is a general rule; however, there are occasionally exceptions to this rule.

The key to distinguishing these two is the pH of the urine. Distal tubular acidosis is the inability to dump hydrogen ions into the urine. Therefore, the presence of an alkaline urine pH, in light of the severity of the acidosis, makes distal tubular acidosis the most likely diagnosis.[35]

---

[35] Distal renal tubular acidosis results in nephrocalcinosis. If they note increased echogenicity on renal ultrasound, this would be another indication that distal renal tubular acidosis is the diagnosis.

376) B) The clinical scenario described is that of nephrotic syndrome, and since **minimal change nephrotic syndrome is the most common cause of nephrotic syndrome, this is the most likely diagnosis**. Focal segmental glomerulonephritis is the second most common cause of nephrotic syndrome. Lupus nephritis is a disease more common in adolescents, not in a child of 4. Therefore, it is important to pay attention to the age of the child presented when considering the differential diagnosis.

There is nothing in the vignette to indicate liver failure or a diagnosis of Henoch-Schönlein purpura.

377) B) Given the alkaline pH of the urine, the most likely etiology is proteus since proteus contains an enzyme that produces ammonia from urea. An additional finding they could describe would be a "foul odor".

378) D) All of the choices can be associated with and/or result in hemolytic uremic syndrome **with the exception of an X-linked recessive inheritance pattern**. Indeed, both oral contraceptives and pregnancy can result in hemolytic uremic syndrome.

There is an inheritance pattern associated with hemolytic uremic syndrome, but it is an **autosomal recessive or dominant**, not an X-linked inheritance pattern. You should consider this choice if they present you with a classic case of hemolytic uremic syndrome presenting in siblings over a period of time. If you really want to get technical,[36] it is believed that the inherited form of hemolytic uremic syndrome is due to *Factor H deficiency* of the "alternative pathway" of complement.[37]

379) C) The most ominous sign of glomerular disease is casts containing RBCs, not serrated or dysmorphic RBCs. The presence of dysmorphic RBCs does, however, *suggest* glomerular disease, but *the absence does not rule it out*. Regarding choice E, a "spot" urine calcium/creatinine check is sufficient to rule out hypercalciuria as a cause of hematuria; a 24-hour sample is not needed.

---

[36] Or want to score high and not just pass like the rest of us.

[37] Whatever that is; I can hardly remember the "traditional" pathway of complement, let alone the alternative. I would look it up except the cloud of dust enveloping the book might trigger a hyperacute case of hemolytic uremic syndrome right on the spot, and it isn't worth the risk.

380) D) Calcium, Oxalate, struvite and cystine can be seen on plain film x-ray.; uric acid stones cannot.

Cystine stones are only faintly radiopaque but this is the boards.

381) C) Helical nonenhanced CT is superior to IVP and other studies in offering the highest sensitivity and specificity in identifying small stones. Other diagnoses in the differential likewise can be identified with this study.

382) A) Recurrent nephrolithiasis is the only clinical manifestation of cystinuria, However in addition to cystine stones it can, albeit rarely, be associated with calcium oxalate stones.

Treatment includes increased fluid intake and alkalinization of urine.

Cystinuria is distinct form cystinosis which is a lysosomal storage disease which is not associated with renal stones.

383) E) Oligohydramnios and bilateral hydronephrosis would be consistent with prune belly syndrome and posterior urethral valves. Note that posterior urethral valves are more common and would be correct if you had to make one choice only.

384) B) Oral steroids are used in other forms of nephrotic syndrome but not in congenital nephrotic syndrome.

High protein diets are used to offset urinary protein loss. ACE inhibitors are used to reduce protein loss. Thyroxine would be used to offset thyroid-binding globulin. Low dose aspirin is used to prevent hypercoagulability due to the loss of protein anti-clotting factors.

385) D) Hypertension in a teenager needs to be addressed. Since the elevated blood pressure was documented on 3 separate occasions by 3 different nurses, by definition hypertension exists. The best initial treatment is weight loss often with a nutrition consult and exercise.

Rheumatology

386) C) Penicillin G or VK, sulfisoxazole, sulfadiazine, sulfonamides in general as well as erythromycin can all be used for preventing rheumatic fever recurrence. Cefaclor PO a 3rd generation cephalosporin would not be effective treatment for recurrent rheumatic fever.

387) C) Recognizing that the cardiac manifestations are the most serious ones, you have probably narrowed your choices down to B and C. If you have not focused on details you will have a 50% chance of answering this incorrectly.

Remember, mitral valve insufficiency will often be the initial or only manifestation during an initial attack. However only 30% of children will have any evidence of it a year later.

On the other hand, when **aortic insufficiency** occurs, it leads to permanent damage in 90% of cases.

Therefore the most important long term concern will be aortic insufficiency rather than mitral valve insufficiency

Rheumatic fever *never* causes *permanent* joint damage. If they state that there is a rapid relief of symptoms with salicylate administration, this is typical and a dead give away in the wording of the question. If they describe joint pain continuing past the acute phase, then the questioner is leading you to a different diagnosis.

Sydenham's chorea can last up to 15 weeks at most. The typical erythema marginatum rash is short lived.

388) C) High persistent fever is the earliest sign, which makes it a difficult disorder to diagnose before the other signs manifest. The fever remits with treatment with IVIG and high dose aspirin.

389) D) Erythema infectiosum is another name for "Fifth Disease" which is another name for "Slap Cheek Disease" caused by Parvovirus B19. Slap yourself on the cheek if you answer this easy question incorrectly.

Erythema marginatum is the rash that is one of the major Jones criteria.

390) 1) (C)
2) (F)
3) (D)
4) (B)
5) (E)
6) (A)

A WBC count less than 200 would be consistent with normal synovial fluid. Trauma would result in joint effusion with synovial fluid with more WBC than normal and increased viscosity and clear.

Decreased viscosity with roughly 5,000 WBC and cloudy would be consistent with a diagnosis of rheumatic fever.

JRA would present with a synovial fluid, which is cloudy with decreased viscosity with a markedly elevated WBC in the 20,000 range

Septic arthritis would present with synovial fluid which is yellow, decreased viscosity and very high WBC in the 200,000 range

Kendall Jackson chardonnay is fluid like septic arthritis is yellow, with bouquet with a kick and a slight after-taste, 10,000 + epithelial cells and maybe a handful of WBC's

391) 1) (E)
2) (A)
3) (B)
4) (C)
5) (D)

Mixed connective tissue disease is associated with high titers of antibodies to an RNase-sensitive component of extractable nuclear antigen. It has some clinical features in common with JRA, SLE, and scleroderma.

In *antiphospholipid syndrome*, there are antibodies to phospholipids that cross-react with the spirochete antigen. This is the explanation for the false-positive VDRL.

Wegener's granulomatosis is due to a systemic vasculitis.

Schönlein-Henoch purpura is a result of vasculitis that is IgA mediated. When the kidneys are involved, the histopathology is identical to Berger's disease (IgA nephropathy).

Although anti-SM is only found in 30% of patients with *SLE*, when it is positive it is a reliable confirmation of a diagnosis of SLE.

392) C) While all of the choices are consistent with a variety of conditions that include hypermobility syndrome, including choice E, which is a description of William's syndrome,[38] the vast majority of children with hypermobility syndrome have no other conditions and will not be noted by their pediatrician.

393) D) Patients with **systemic lupus erythematosus** typically have anemia of chronic illness. However they can also have an autoimmune hemolytic anemia. Immune mediated thrombocytopenia also occurs. Leukopenia is not uncommon.

However leukocytosis is not typically seen in lupus.

---

[38] Easy to remember if you use the zany characters actor Robin Williams portrays as your mnemonic.

394) B) Neonatal lupus erythematosus is due to transplacental transfer of antibodies which can result in cutaneous lupus lesions which resolve without scarring. Hepatitis is another possible manifestation which resolves as the maternal antibodies disappear.

However congenital heart block is irreversible because it is due to permanent damage to the conducting system making placement of a permanent pacemaker necessary.

395) C) Non steroidal anti inflammatory medications are used to treat arthritis and fever in patients with lupus. Glucocorticosteroid are used in particular to treat renal, hematological, and CNS manifestations.

Sunscreen is important to protect against cutaneous manifestations. Cyclophosphamide is used particularly for renal and CNS manifestations

Insulin is not used in treating lupus.

Substance Abuse

396) C) Alcohol; had they asked, "What is the most widely used *illegal* drug?" the answer would have been marijuana.

Some might argue that love is the most widely used drug but it is not a registered trademark nor is it controlled by the DEA, as of this printing at least.

397) B) The physical findings are due to amphetamine which is adrenergic. This would explain the increased blood pressure, heart rate and the dilated pupils (**mydriasis**) and abdominal cramping

There is nothing in the history to suggest undiagnosed bipolar disease. Alcohol and cannabis abuse would not present with this clinical history.

PCP abuse might present with tachycardia and hypertension but they would also need to describe hallucinations and/or slurred speech to distinguish from amphetamine abuse.

398) C) The patient is presenting with acute intoxication secondary to PCP and marijuana.

The clinical presentation of PCP intoxication depends on the degree of intoxication

Low dose – mild inebriation

Moderate dose – catatonic blank stare, muscle rigidity, hypertension and tachycardia

Large doses – coma, seizure and respiratory distress

This patient is presenting with symptoms of moderate dose intoxication. The muscle rigidity can lead to rhabdomyolysis. If serum myoglobin is high enough there is a risk for deposition in the renal tubules causing renal toxicity

Therefore the correct answer is to measure serum myoglobin.

Rectal Valium would not be a good idea in a patient who is catatonic with muscle rigidity for what should be obvious reasons. However IV Valium to relax the patient might not be a bad idea but was not one of the listed choices.

399) D) Drug use among high school students was at its highest in the 1970's this was followed by a decline in the 80's and then a gradual increase in the 1990's

Cigarette smoking among 8th -12th graders has *decreased* over the past decade.

The use of performance enhancing drugs *increases* the likelihood of use of other illicit drugs. Inhalant abuse is more prevalent among 8th graders than 12th graders

Among other risk factors for substance abuse alienation from conventional norms is one of them. Therefore homosexual adolescents have rates of substance abuse that are significantly higher than heterosexual peers.

400) D) High pitched voice, gynecomastia and pustular – papular acne would be a result of anabolic steroid abuse. The mood swings and mania would also be part of the presentation.

Growth hormone would not present with acne or the aggressive behavior depicted in this vignette.

Notes

_____

_____

_____

_____

_____

_____

_____

_____

_____

_____

_____

_____

Notes

Notes